THE DEVIL'S MIRACLE

Opain was the ultimate miracle drug. A few doses and a woman was totally protected from pain.

Laniet Teague could testify to that.

She had been given Opain and no longer did she fear pain at all. Quite the reverse.

In a dingy Greenwich Village apartment, she told the bearded, motorcycle-jacketed man who had picked her up that he and any of his friends could do anything they wanted with her . . . use her . . . abuse her . . . whip her if they liked . . . as long as their strength and her flesh could take it.

Laniet Teague was one of the first of the women to be freed of pain—and turned into a slave of something far more agonizing . . . the ultimate sick desire. . . .

PAIN

More Bestsellers From SIGNET

PAIN

Michael Carson

A SIGNET BOOK
NEW AMERICAN LIBRARY
TIMES MIRROR

PUBLISHER'S NOTE

This novel is a work of fiction. Names, characters, places, and incidents are either the product of the author's imagination or are used fictitiously, and any resemblance to actual persons, living or dead, events, or locales is entirely coincidental.

 SIGNET TRADEMARK REG. U.S. PAT. OFF. AND FOREIGN COUNTRIES
REGISTERED TRADEMARK—MARCA REGISTRADA
HECHO EN CHICAGO, U.S.A.

SIGNET, SIGNET CLASSICS, MENTOR, PLUME, MERIDIAN AND NAL BOOKS *are published by The New American Library, Inc., 1633 Broadway, New York, New York 10019*

FIRST PRINTING, AUGUST, 1982

1 2 3 4 5 6 7 8 9

PRINTED IN THE UNITED STATES OF AMERICA

For Judy, who loved every word.
And for Shelly Lowenkopf, who didn't.

Special thanks to Hilary Ross, my editor, Phyllis Westberg, my agent, and Dennis Lynds, Chuck Gates, and John B. MacDonald, for their inspiration.

1

"Got any aspirin, Pete?"

"Top drawer on the left," Dr. Peterson said, barely glancing up from the charred and twisted body of the young woman on the autopsy table. He rolled a sliced crescent of the woman's adrenal gland between his gloved fingers, studied the tiny hemorrhages which mottled its surface. "Should be the other way around," he said.

"What should?" Dr. Ames washed down the two aspirin with a swig of coffee, pulled on his gloves, and approached the table.

"I've been up working all night, and you've got the headache," Peterson said.

Ames nodded, took the piece of adrenal gland which Peterson handed him. "My wife's birthday," he said. "I should know by now I can't drink champagne."

Peterson stepped back from the table and relit his cigar stub, then stripped off his blood-smeared gloves and sat heavily on the stool at the dictation counter.

"Jesus, what a mess," Ames said, seeming to have just noticed the girl on the table. "What happened?"

"Set herself on fire and jumped out of a fifth-floor apartment window. Like a Roman candle."

Ames began to sew up the gaping opening in the dead

woman's chest and abdomen. "Drugs," he said, shaking his head.

Peterson leaned back against the green counter and poured the dregs of last night's coffee into his cup. "No drugs," he said. "She's clean."

"What, then? Even a severe depression wouldn't go out this way."

Peterson tasted his coffee, made a face, and slowly got to his feet. "Her parents are coming up from Scranton. Said the only thing she'd ever had trouble with was a tennis elbow. Twenty-two years old, well-adjusted, happy, no depression."

"That's what they all say."

Peterson nodded his agreement.

"Anything except the adrenal hemorrhage?" Ames asked.

"Same thing in the stomach. The colon. And brain. Everything else seems to be from the fall or the burns."

Ames worked silently for a while. "Doesn't make sense," he said. "Stress hemorrhages. From what?"

"No good reason for them. No infection. Nothing to suggest severe pain. No history of anything."

"You wouldn't commit suicide over a little elbow hurt," Ames said. "Can you imagine the pain she must have felt coming out of that window? On fire?"

Peterson caught himself staring at the young woman's distorted right arm, obscenely bent the wrong way, as if trying to serve a tennis ball from behind her back. He walked to her side and gently straightened her arm to its normal position, trying to ignore the grating sounds of bone and sinew as it resisted his efforts. Suddenly it snapped into place, and the cold, stark room became oppressive. Stale. He turned to leave. At the door, he looked back at the lifeless girl on the stainless-steel table, somehow relieved that her arm was again pointing in the right direction. "Whatever it was," he said, "it can't hurt her anymore."

Jennifer Barton glanced out her apartment window to see a misty January rain collecting on her fire escape, the drops hanging as though reluctant to fall, but uncertain whether to freeze. The early-morning traffic three floors below snarled as work-bound New Yorkers honked impatiently and fought to escape the congestion. She moved her African violet from the windowsill to the counter in her tiny kitchen, and probed its soil with her finger. It didn't need water, but obviously didn't like the cold chill seeping through the windowpanes. She rinsed her finger under the tap, and spoke to her two fringetail goldfish. "Good morning, Sushi. Saki." She tapped her fingernails lightly against the round glass bowl. The fish immediately lined themselves up to face her, little gold soldiers, their mouths working silently.

"This is for you, Sushi," she said, dropping a single pellet of food into the far corner of the bowl for the larger fish. Quickly crushing another pellet between two spoons, Jennifer sprinkled the food at the opposite end of the bowl for the smaller fish. "Hurry, Saki," she said, watching to be sure the little one got its share. She repeated the maneuver, delighted that Saki had finally learned to get his food while the larger Sushi was fully occupied.

"I'll change your water tonight," she promised as she hurried to answer the phone.

"It's Aunt Tilda, Jennie. The flowers you sent were beautiful." The familiar Southern-accented voice held the slight tremor of advancing age.

"Happy birthday, Aunt Tilda. How's the weather in Atlanta?"

"It's always cold when you're seventy-three."

Jennifer listened as her only living relative talked about the weather, her health, and day-to-day problems of great significance to her.

"People just can't live on Social Security, with the price of groceries and all. I know you're a doctor now, and young, but you put something aside for your old age, Jennie."

Jennifer sat on the arm of the chair beside the phone. She sensed the old woman's loneliness, and made an extra effort to cheer her up. "Aunt Tilda, I've been thinking.

I'd like to send you a little money each month. I can't send much. Not yet. But a little something to help out."

Her aunt made a minimal protest, then agreed that maybe fifty dollars a month would be real nice. "You're just like your dear mother, Jennie. She was always doing for people. I've never really gotten over . . . well, when she passed on."

Jennifer listened to Tilda's sobs for a moment, then changed the subject in an effort to improve her aunt's mood. "I start my new job today, and I'm really looking forward to it."

Aunt Tilda seemed to hesitate for a moment, as though reluctant to adjust to the happy tone. "Is that the plastic surgery?"

"Not yet," Jennifer replied. "I'll work in the pain clinic for a while. Then I start my plastic fellowship."

Tilda started to say something, but stopped. Her voice contained more of a question than her words when she asked, "How much longer, Jennie?"

Jennifer felt her back straighten, her muscles tense. "Only about six months. After I start the fellowship."

The disappointment in her aunt's voice was clear. "It seems so long," she said. "I thought you'd be back long before now. They need good doctors here. Why, you can't get an appointment in less than two weeks."

Jennifer caught herself nodding her understanding, then shook her head. "I'm not quite ready yet. It takes time to specialize."

"I suppose so," the resigned voice answered. "It just seems to me you're putting it off for some reason." After a brief silence, Tilda asked, "Don't you want to go into practice, Jennie?"

Jennifer felt her cheeks heat up. "Of course I do."

"I thought maybe after all you'd been through—"

"I'm fine," Jennifer said quickly. "Really." She glanced at her watch again and stood. "I've got to run, Aunt Tilda. Happy birthday. I love you. And I'll write soon." When she hung up, she exhaled a long breath, dialed the operator back, and asked her to bill the long-distance call to her phone, only vaguely aware of the cool perspiration beading her forehead and upper lip. She wiped her palms on her white uniform skirt and started for the door.

At about the time Jennifer Barton finished talking with her aunt, a terrified Melanie Wardner inched her way across the narrow space from her hospital stretcher to the cold sheets covering the operating table. She closed her eyes as a heavy strap tightened around her hips, and wished she could stop shaking. "Don't hurt me," she said. "Please."

Dr. Bevins took one of her cold hands in his and leaned forward. "You won't feel a thing, Melanie. Dr. Todd is going to give you a shot and you'll go right to sleep." He squeezed her fingers gently.

"You're sure?"

"I promise."

The anesthesiologist quickly pierced the skin of the girl's arm with the intravenous needle. Her body immediately went rigid, and she let out a shrill, ear-splitting scream that reverberated throughout the tiled operating room.

"Dammit, Melanie, it's only a pinprick," the anesthesiologist said, seating and taping the needle into her vein.

Melanie bit her contorted lower lip and perspiration beaded her forehead. "I'm sorry," she sobbed. "I can't stand pain. If you hurt me, I'll die. I know I will." She began to whine as her body shook in racking spasms.

Dr. Todd injected a measured amount of sodium Pentothal into the I.V. tubing and quickly followed it with a bolus of muscle relaxant, succinyl choline. Seconds later, Melanie was fast asleep, limp and unconscious beneath the harsh white lights over the operating table. The surgeon shook his head at Todd's annoyed shrug, his furrowed brow visible in the slit between his green scrub cap and mask. "Now you know why I couldn't do her in the office. She has absolutely no tolerance for pain." The surgeon left the room to scrub his hands as two nurses slid Melanie down toward the foot of the operating table. They lifted her feet and legs into heavy canvas stirrups suspended from steel posts, her rubbery knees separating without resistance, exposing her pubic area to the shadowless beam of the bright lights.

Outside the room, the chief O.R. nurse approached Dr. Bevins as he lathered and scrubbed his hands and arms. "What was all the screaming?"

Bevins tossed the red plastic pick into the scrub sink after cleaning under his nails, and applied a foamy brush to his arms. "That was just from starting the I.V. You'd have thought we were taking out her heart without anesthesia."

The nurse nodded. "How long will you be?"

He turned, elbows dripping, leaving a watery trail behind as he approached the operating room. "Ten minutes. It's only a small urethral stricture."

Inside, Melanie was draped in green sheets, the only thing visible her shaved pubis glaring pinkish-white as Dr. Bevins was put into his gown and gloves and seated himself on a stool between her suspended legs.

"Honeymoon cystitis?" Dr. Todd asked.

"Maybe," Bevins replied, checking the lighted end of the metal cystoscope. "She gets a bladder infection every time she has sex. Probably a stricture."

"A pinched pee tube," Todd said absently.

Bevins inserted the long slender instrument into the orifice of Melanie's urethra and advanced it toward her bladder, watching carefully through the telescopic lens for the expected narrowing of the passage. "Lights off."

The circulating nurse switched off the overhead lights, giving Bevins better contrast and visibility of the glistening pink interior of Melanie's urethra.

"Yep, there it is. Sounds, please." The overhead lights came on instantly. Bevins withdrew the cystoscope and reached for the smallest of the urethral sounds, smooth, curved, shiny stainless-steel probes almost phallic in shape, but smaller and more slender than his gloved fingers. He inserted and removed each of several of the metal sounds up Melanie's urethra, each larger than the one before, gradually dilating the narrowed portion of the tubular passage leading from her bladder. The room was silent as he worked, except for the rhythmic sighing of Melanie's breathing as Dr. Todd pressed the black rubber bag at her side.

"One quick look at the bladder and we're through," Bevins announced moments later. As the lights dimmed again, he reinserted the cystoscope and quickly advanced it past the area of earlier constriction into Melanie's bladder. When he leaned forward, his shoulder brushed against the inside of Melanie's thigh, and the canvas strap suspending her leg slipped from its support. The dead-weight of Melanie's limp leg crashed down onto Bevins' shoulder and arm, abruptly driving the metal instrument inward as Bevins reflexively fought for his balance. He yanked the cystoscope away.

"Goddammit," he shouted. "Fix that damned leg. Lights."

The circulating nurse quickly repositioned Melanie's leg and reattached the canvas strap, apologizing as Bevins glared at her. When he turned his attention back to Melanie, he felt his heart sink. Bright red blood gushed from her urethral orifice and trickled down across her pubis, dripping steadily onto his white shoes, beginning to clot on the shiny operating-room floor.

Quickly irrigating her bladder and reinserting the cystoscope, he saw through the blood what he had hoped beyond belief he would not find. "Prep her abdomen and redrape her." He sighed. "Her bladder's ruptured. We'll have to open her up to repair it."

Dr. Todd stood and moved his anesthesia machine to the head of the table as the nurses quickly detached Melanie from the suspension stirrups and slid her back up the table. "Tell scheduling we'll be about three hours," Todd said to one of the nurses. He stared compassionately at Dr. Bevins and added, "It would have to be this one. With her pain threshold, she'll scream for the next two months."

Dr. Bevins stripped off his bloody gloves and slammed them onto the floor. He opened the door to rescrub, and barked at the circulating nurse, "Call Pain Control. Dr.

Neilson. Tell him to have somebody in Recovery when she wakes up."

Six floors and mazes of hallways below the operating rooms, Laniet Teague sat alone in a barren gray room facing a console of blinking lights and dials that rested on a wooden table only inches away from her. Green, white, yellow, and blue plastic-coated wires extended from her red-haired temples, her fingertips, and her bare toes to the whirring machine. Her wrists were secured by padded straps to the wooden arms of the chair on which she sat, her right arm awkwardly positioned because of a plaster cast, and she held in one hand a heavy gray cord with a raised, central plastic button. She gazed at the digital clocklike screen atop the console, on which appeared the number 24. She felt her mouth spread into a sly smile as she pressed the button again, and felt a searing pain beneath her nails, where the wires attached. Almost simultaneously, she felt a crushing pressure in her head, and saw the dark spots that always came with her migraines. But the headache had gone up to only 19 on the digital readout. She held the button down with a trembling thumb as pain screamed along her nail beds and up the nerves of her arms and legs to her brain. The number 26 came on the screen as she felt the beginnings of the sensation she craved. A soft, undulating wave of softness swept over her, as though she were wrapped in a fleecy cloud, or floating in a sea of tepid Jell-O. Perspiration trickled down her nose and stung her eyes, suddenly feeling like droplets of morning dew on roses, or a fresh spring rain. What had felt like a constricting steel band around her head moments earlier, ever tightening, had become a soft cloth soaked in ancient healing herbs that caressed and soothed her mind and her pain. She pressed harder with her thumb, and watched anxiously as the number rose to 28, and the pain became so intense, and the pleasure so great, it was almost more than she could bear. She was hardly aware of the pounding of her heart against her ribs, or of her labored breathing as the red numbers and the console began to spin before her eyes.

She fought at the edge of consciousness to press the button harder and harder, and floated lazily into a vast darkness just before the control slipped from her grasp and fell to the floor. Moments later, Laniet Teague was carefully unstrapped from the heavy chair and lifted effortlessly by wide, thick hands that carried her through a nearby door. Perspiration-drenched but smiling, she dreamed of Jell-O seas and cotton clouds and morning dew as she was placed on a high bed at the end of a dim corridor and secured in place with leather restraints around her wrists and ankles.

2

—————•◦•═◦═•◦•—————

Jennifer grabbed her purse and sweater and took the creaky elevator down to subbasement level, where she entered the underground tunnel that led to the cavernous New Hope University Hospital. Her heels echoed in the dank catacomblike passage, devoid of the usual hordes of uniformed hospital personnel, causing her to glance at her watch. Five to nine. She'd make it right on time. She bounded up two flights of stairs to the first floor, raced past the locked doors of the old hospital morgue, and rounded the corner toward the Pain Control Clinic, suddenly aware of the sterile hospital smells of alcohol sponges and disinfectants.

Several patients sat on wooden clinic benches in front of the reception desk, glancing curiously at her white uniform as she slowed to a more dignified walk. The nurse behind the desk ignored her presence until she spoke. "Excuse me."

The nurse looked up without expression, her blond hair neatly tucked under her white cap. The hair didn't match her dark eyebrows. She was almost a head taller than Jennifer when she straightened, probably five-seven or five-eight in shoes, and at least ten years older. Pushing forty. Her brown eyes were questioning.

"I'm Dr. Barton," Jennifer began. "I'm to work with Dr. Neilson."

"Clinic started a half-hour ago," the nurse said.

Jennifer glanced at her watch again. "But it's only nine o'clock. The schedule said—"

"We start at eight-thirty. Promptly. Dr. Neilson sets his own hours."

Jennifer glanced at the nurse's name tag. It said "Kane." She forced herself to smile. "You're Miss Kane?"

The woman nodded curtly. "Nurse Kane. I'll show you where you'll work." She turned and led the way down a short hallway to a cluster of examining rooms.

Inside the first room, Jennifer saw a standard paper-covered vinyl examining table, stethoscope, blood-pressure cuff, percussion hammer, and small desk and metal stool. Nurse Kane picked up a clipboard from the desk. "This is our history form. It's more detailed than usual, and must be completed on every patient. Each patient is assigned a number, to be recorded on the top line."

Jennifer recoiled slightly. There was no space for a name.

"Your only interest is the medical history," Kane said. "Past illnesses. Present illnesses. Particularly descriptions of pain. Type, severity, frequency, detailed descriptions of painful sensations, and how the pain responded to medications. Any history of allergies to medications is essential. Do a complete physical on each patient, and record your working diagnosis. Do not order any medications on your own."

Jennifer felt her earlobes begin to burn. She flipped through the pages of the detailed history form and determined not to lose her temper. She set the form on the desk. "Perhaps I should meet Dr. Neilson before I begin."

Nurse Kane replaced the loose pages in the clipboard. "He's in his lab this morning, then seeing hospital consults. He'll be in clinic this afternoon. I'll get your first patient."

Jennifer let out a long sigh as Nurse Kane left, and

walked into the hall to check the adjacent exam rooms. There was an identical room to her left, and two rooms across the hall. The door to one room across the hall was closed. She pushed it open for a quick look before her patient arrived, and heard a resounding crash and clatter as the door thudded against something inside.

"Jesus H. Christ," a heavy male voice bellowed. "What do you think you're doing?"

Jennifer jumped, startled, and looked up into a pair of dark eyes blazing with anger and accusation. A quick look told her she had knocked over a medication table, with syringes and glass vials still tumbling from the table and rolling across the vinyl-tiled floor. "I'm sorry." She slipped through the half-open door and bent to pick up the vials.

"Just get out. And learn to knock next time."

She straightened instantly, her cheeks fiery hot, certain she had flushed blood-red. As she did, her shoulder painfully caught the edge of the table, tossing its remaining contents to the floor. She scrambled to catch the falling vials, and felt glass crunch beneath her feet as she stepped on others rolling across the floor. The man in the white lab coat glared down at her, hands on hips, his head shaking from side to side.

Jennifer stood absolutely still, at a loss for words, humiliated, and placed the one glass vial she had retrieved back on the righted table. She forced her chin high. "I'm sorry. I'll pay for any damage." And she turned and crunched her way out the door.

Nurse Kane turned from the patient she directed into the adjacent examination room, glanced toward the jumbled mess behind Jennifer, and let out a short, judgmental sigh. "Your first patient is waiting, doctor."

Jennifer tried to avoid her eyes and walked straight toward the exam room. "Was that Dr. Neilson?"

"Dr. West. And lucky for you."

Jennifer closed the door behind her, and extended her hand to an elderly woman seated on the exam table. The chart identified the patient as number 1024. "I'm Dr.

Barton," Jennifer said, still aware of her own rapid pulse in her ears.

"Why can't you people do something about this pain?" the woman grumbled, ignoring Jennifer's outstretched hand.

Jennifer saw the anguish and hostility in the woman's eyes. They were old eyes, tired. They'd seen it all, mostly unkind and without hope. The woman's faded scarf outlined a gaunt face, heavily lined and uncared-for. Her frayed overcoat was stained and misshapen above canary legs clad in opaque brown stockings, like too many coats of heavy paint. Jennifer sat behind the small desk and read through the woman's chart. The history and physical forms were complete, and the diagnosis was shingles.

"Did you have chickenpox as a child?" Jennifer asked.

"I already answered that a dozen times."

Jennifer glanced through the rest of the woman's chart. Under "medications" she saw only the number 1024 recorded each week for six weeks. She had no idea what medications the woman had been given. She stood, frustrated and angry. "Excuse me," she said, and left the room.

At the reception desk, Nurse Kane seemed annoyed to see her so soon. "I can't tell you what medication she's on," Kane replied. "She's getting whatever the computer instructed. It's part of the study Dr. Neilson is doing."

"But it isn't working," Jennifer said. "Shingles is very painful, and whatever she's on isn't helping. She needs something stronger."

"Then you record that in the chart. Just that the medication hasn't helped her pain."

"I'd like to ask Dr. Neilson to give her something else. It's been six weeks."

"She will be given drug 1024, vial number seven. Those are Dr. Neilson's orders. I'll have Dr. West quantify her pain. You may as well watch, and learn how it's done."

Jennifer followed the rigid nurse down the hall and watched as the old woman, Mrs. 1024, sat in front of an

array of instruments like a TV control booth and allowed Nurse Kane to attach wires to her temples and
fingertips. Moments later, Dr. West emerged from his
exam room and took the seat beside the patient. He
glanced at Jennifer but didn't speak. If he hadn't been so
nasty, Jennifer would have thought him attractive in an
animalistic sort of way. His hair was so black it shone,
the color of a raven preening in the sun, and his brows
were heavy and full. His nose was straight and strong,
and his jaw angled almost square. His shoulders were
broad above narrow hips, and his arms long as he
reached out to touch the woman's hand.

"You know how this works, Mary," he said in a
smooth, deep tone.

The old woman nodded. Dr. West turned a dial on
the control panel, and Jennifer saw Mary flinch slightly
and twist her wrinkled mouth in silence. The number 6
appeared on the digital panel above the dials. The
woman shook her head without speaking, her tired old
eyes focused somewhere in the distance. West turned the
dial farther to the right. She shook her head again. When
the number 8 appeared on the screen, Mary grunted,
nodded abruptly, and said, "That's it. That's the same
pain."

West flipped a switch which extinguished the lighted
panels on the console, and removed the plastic-coated
wires from the patient. "The same as last week, Mary.
But it's better than before."

"Humph," she snorted. "Don't feel any better. For all
the good you're doing me, I might as well take an aspirin."

West smiled and patted the old woman's hand. "You
know the rules, Mary. You can't take any other medicine while you're under treatment. Nurse Kane will give
you your injection."

Jennifer wasn't sure exactly what West had done with
the complex machine, but she suspected he was measuring the patient's level of pain from her shingles. She
knew that shingles was a blisterlike eruption along the
nerves, usually around the rib cage, and caused by the

chickenpox virus. It was supposed to be very painful, and sometimes persisted for weeks or months. But the old woman didn't seem to be in great pain. At least she didn't show it.

After Nurse Kane gave the injection and Mary left, Jennifer walked to the reception desk to ask Nurse Kane how the machine worked.

"Dr. Neilson has determined the average pain levels of hundreds of illnesses. The electrodes to the fingers deliver an electrical stimulus direct to the pain receptors, the nerve endings. When patients have pain in another part of the body, they can ignore the pain in their fingers until it reaches the same intensity. When the stimulus just cancels out the other pain, we know how strong the original pain is."

Nurse Kane's unemotional explanation was interrupted by a nervous, pale woman of about fifty with puffy eyelids and broken capillaries dotting her cheeks and nose. Jennifer could smell cheap wine on the woman's breath when she spoke around a crumpled handkerchief clutched to her mouth.

"I'm looking for my daughter, Laniet Teague. Is she here?"

Nurse Kane considered the woman for a moment. "There's nobody here by that name."

"But she's been coming here," the woman said. "She's got red hair, about my height. A pretty girl."

"She isn't here."

"She said she's been here twice a week all month. This is the pain clinic?"

Kane nodded, and started to turn away.

"Please, nurse. Laniet didn't come home all week. She's run off before, but I have to know. She's got migraine headaches something terrible. And she broke her arm last week. She may be hurtin' real bad."

Nurse Kane took a deep breath and opened her appointment book. "What did you say her name was?"

"Teague. Laniet Teague. A pretty girl. Twenty-three. Red hair."

Kane flipped the pages impatiently. "There's no Laniet

Teague in the book. You must be mistaken. She's never been here."

Jennifer saw the woman's chin tremble slightly as her eyes went dull and distant. She removed her veined, liver-spotted hand from the desk where she had rested it, slightly nodded, and walked slowly away.

"Why don't you go to lunch now," Nurse Kane said abruptly. "I'll test you on the pain-threshold stimulator before Dr. Neilson arrives at one o'clock. So you'll understand what you're doing. Be back by twelve-thirty."

As Jennifer walked down to the hospital cafeteria, Laniet Teague opened her eyes and tried to focus on the gray walls of the desolate room. She shifted her hips on the hard bed, hearing a slight rustle and crinkling of the plastic mattress cover beneath her, but the leather restraints on her wrists and ankles kept her from turning onto her side. She searched with her right thumb for the magic button, but felt only the cold steel of the bed's side rails. She took a great deep breath and exhaled slowly, then turned her gaze to the plaster cast on her arm. By straining hard against the straps on her arms and legs, she was able to shift toward the right side of the narrow bed, where she tentatively swung the plaster cast against the side rail with a dull thud. She immediately felt the jolt of pain in her arm, like an electric shock, from where the edges of the jagged bones scraped together. She closed her eyes for a moment, waiting for the sensation to fully register in her brain, and felt her heart begin to race in her chest. She slowly shifted her arm and shoulder up in the air as far as the restraints would allow, and slammed her casted arm down against the side rail again, the heavy thunk followed by a brief harmonic sound of vibrating metal. Beads of sweat trickled from her armpits toward her back, causing a slight involuntary shudder to gallop through her. She heard distant footsteps beyond the door, and a clicking sound as the latch opened. She closed her eyes and feigned sleep, forcing her breathing to slow until the latch clicked again and the footsteps receded. As she lay waiting, she absently twisted her wrist in the restraints, aware of a slight delicious tingling as the strap rubbed its way deep into her flesh.

Jennifer Barton waited impatiently in the long hospital cafeteria line and tried to guess who worked in which department. She decided the three talkative girls ahead of her were delivery-room nurses, in their short blue scrub dresses and white coats. The haggard young man with a day's growth of beard had to be an intern, and left his full tray of food on the counter when his beeper sounded in the dessert section. She paid for her tuna salad and tea and searched for a table of friendly faces to join. Everybody seemed fully occupied with food and enthusiastic conversations. One gray-haired nurse stubbed out a cigarette and vacated a tiny table in a nearby corner as Jennifer approached, so she took the empty seat and sat alone, feeling mildly conspicuous in the buzzing room.

As she began to eat, she recognized one face across the room, Dr. West, from the clinic that morning. He seemed totally engrossed in an animated discussion with a pretty dark-haired nurse whose white uniform was short enough to show off long shapely legs discreetly crossed, one foot rhythmically swinging beneath the table. He seemed to be doing all the talking. West appeared to glance toward Jennifer once, and she smiled automatically, but sensed no response on his part as he thumped his palm against the distant table to make some point. Jennifer concentrated on her tuna salad and wished she had brought along something to read.

When she finished her lunch, she stood, swung the strap of her leather bag over one shoulder, and turned to carry her tray to the conveyor belt for dirty dishes. Suddenly her tray jostled out of her grasp and clattered noisily to the floor, the teacup shattering into a thousand flying fragments as the plastic plate bounced under a nearby table.

"Still being a klutz, I see," Dr. West said.

Jennifer instinctively grabbed a napkin to wipe dripping coffee from his white coat. "I didn't see you. I'm so sorry."

He grasped her wrist and took the napkin from her hand. "Maybe I'd better do that," he grumbled. "You'd manage some way to make it worse."

She felt her cheeks heat up instantly, but stooped to pick up his spilled Styrofoam cup and her tray.

"Nice legs," he said. "That's something."

She quickly turned her exposed knees away from him, put the available pieces of broken teacup on the tray with his cup, and stood, her blood boiling. As she started to maneuver past him, West reached out for the tray, grinning.

"You can either get out of my way," Jennifer said in as calm a voice as she could muster, "or wear this tray on your cocky head." With that, and ignoring his look of amused compliance, she shouldered her way past him, had to stop and turn back when she realized she had gone in the wrong direction. She didn't look at West as she hurried by, her cheeks aflame.

Tossing the tray among others on the conveyor, Jennifer quickly surveyed the large room and picked her way between crowded tables toward the nearest exit. Just as she reached the outside hall, a firm but gentle hand took her arm.

"Hey," West said. "I'm sorry."

"You should be." She started to turn away.

"I really am," he persisted. When she looked up at him, the arrogant grin she expected wasn't there. He appeared quite sincere, the way he had been when he spoke with the patient with shingles in the clinic.

"It's okay," Jennifer said, her anger level falling.

He extended his hand. "I'm David West. And I didn't mean to come on so strong this morning."

She hesitated for an instant, made her decision, and shook his hand. "Jennifer Barton," she said.

West smiled, looked at his watch. "It's too early for clinic. Can I buy you a cup of coffee?"

Jennifer started to say no, to make an excuse, but

something in his tone of voice convinced her otherwise. "Tea," she said, and walked back inside.

West got their respective drinks and joined her at the table. "I didn't mean to appear cocky," he said.

She considered him for a moment. "And I'm not usually such a klutz."

He smiled again, a genuine smile. "Truce?"

She laughed and nodded. "Truce, David West." She sipped at her tea.

"What brings you to the House of Hurt?" he asked.

She didn't understand.

"The Pain Control Clinic."

"Oh. It's temporary. I'm waiting for a fellowship in plastic surgery. I'm ENT and head and neck."

West nodded. "I'm neurosurgery. My last year. Where'd you train?"

"Jefferson Medical. In Philadelphia."

"You don't sound native. Is that Southern I hear?"

Jennifer smiled. "Atlanta. I thought I'd lost it."

West sipped at his coffee, tilted his chair back. "Well, you've met the charming and gregarious Rachel Kane. How do you like it so far?"

Jennifer shrugged. "Too early to tell. It's not something I'd want to do forever."

"Me neither. I'm there because our department requires a research project before finishing the residency. I'm only around two or three days a week." He looked questioningly at her and waited.

"I need the money. And it's the only way I could get staff housing."

"Where'd they put you?"

"Brigton House. Across the street."

"I'm in Hanover House. The tall building known as Peyton Place. How does the pain clinic tie in with ENT or plastic?"

She toyed with the Styrofoam cup, pressing her fingernails into little crescent patterns in its soft surface. "One—ears, noses, and throats and plastic-surgery patients experience pain. Two—it was the only job available till I start my fellowship. What's Neilson like?"

West paused to respond to a greeting from a tall, dreamy-eyed blond nurse who ran her fingertips along his shoulder as she said hello. The nurse gave Jennifer an appraising glance and swayed away. West didn't appear to be concerned. "He's not bad," West said, "if you like obsessive geniuses. He's totally hung up on his 'Neilson ratings,' forgive the pun. Kidney colic is a Neilson thirty-two. Tooth abscesses are eighteens. Shingles runs from eight to fourteen."

"It's a unique idea. I've never heard of anybody measuring pain before. Things either hurt a little or a lot."

"But some people hurt a lot with a pain that others would call a little. Their threshold is lower. Same pain, bigger hurt."

The stoic face of the old woman with shingles flashed across Jennifer's memory. "How strong is an eight?"

West wrinkled his forehead. "More than a strep throat, less than having your tonsils out. About like a thrombosed hemorrhoid."

"That hurts."

"It all does. Neilson's after the perfect pain pill. Or shot. The ideal analgesic. One that will magically raise anybody's threshold of pain to the exact level to control, whatever they have. Had your tonsils out? Take a number ten Neilson pill. Got a brain tumor? Number sixteen."

"You don't sound impressed."

West shrugged with his hands. "It's not a bad idea. I just prefer surgery. If a brain tumor hurts or an aneurysm leaks, cut it out or sew it up. I like to see what I'm treating."

Jennifer set her cup down. "Not every painful disease can be cut out, doctor." She was surprised at the sudden edge in her voice.

"Sounds like I touched a nerve."

She studied him for a moment, decided he hadn't intended the pun. "The classic surgeon's personality," she said without sarcasm. "Impatient. Instant diagnoses and solutions. Immediate gratification."

West nodded. "Diagnosed like a true surgeon." He grinned. "What's your recommended treatment?"

Jennifer hesitated, then spoke softly. "I haven't found one." She took a deep breath. "I've tried to correct my own impulsiveness. Without much success, I'm afraid."

"It probably makes you a damned good surgeon. Or at least it's what attracted you to surgery in the first place."

"Maybe," she admitted, then looked up from her cup. "Have you ever experienced real pain, David?"

He narrowed his eyes. "No. Not the kind I think you mean." After a pause he asked, "Have you?"

Jennifer glanced at her watch. Twelve-thirty. She stood quickly and gathered her purse. "I'm due back at the clinic. Nurse Kane wants to put me on the machine before Neilson arrives."

West walked out to the hall with her. "Don't be afraid to admit when it hurts. Kane gets her jollies turning up the dials." He laughed. "I bet she's into S-M, if she can find anybody to play."

As Jennifer approached the hallway into the Pain Control Clinic, Nurse Kane walked out quickly beside a tall, slender man in a white coat with heavy black-rimmed glasses on an aquiline nose. The silver in his striped tie matched the sheen of his temples and sideburns, slightly incongruous with the rest of his dark hair and youthful face. Mid-forties, she guessed. Kane stopped him at Jennifer's side.

"Dr. Neilson has an emergency consult in seventh-floor recovery room. Go with him and complete the history forms." Kane handed Jennifer the familiar sheets. And to Dr. Neilson she said, "I'll get the experiments set up."

Jennifer almost ran to keep up with Neilson, introducing herself on the elevator. His smile and handshake were warm, and his eyes alert and sensitive, though he appeared slightly preoccupied. When they left the elevator, Jennifer felt a jolt of adrenaline flood her system from the incredibly piercing shrieks of agony that came from behind the closed doors to the recovery room.

Inside, glass-shattering screams seemed to bounce off the green walls of the fluorescent-lit room, each new expression of agony beginning almost before the echoes of the last one had died. Of the twenty-odd beds in the long room, six frantic nurses hovered over the bed from which the pathetic cries came. Neilson quickly and silently grabbed the chart from the patient's bed, and scanned the pages.

"No allergies?" he asked, shouting above the girl's incessant cries.

A short-haired nurse near the patient's head responded first, her green scrub suit damp under her arms. "No. She's had a hundred of Demerol and twenty-five of Phenergan. Hasn't touched her."

Jennifer had the desire to cover her ears as the unnerving shrieks grew crescendolike from the small frantic girl who fought with arms and legs pinned awkwardly by the restraining nurses. The girl shook her head violently from side to side, her brown hair whipping across her contorted face. Imprints of a set of fingernails blanched the skin of one arm as a nurse lost her grip and fought to recapture the girl's flailing arm. The nurse's red face was openly hostile, her mouth pinched, eyes narrowed to slits. Dr. Neilson removed a vial from the pocket of his white coat, opened a sterile syringe on the table near her bedside, and drew up the contents of the glass vial. He deftly inserted the needle into the I.V. tubing and began to press the plunger, injecting the medication into the girl's bloodstream. He paused several times, studying his wristwatch, and continued the injections. After what seemed an eternity, but could have been only a few minutes, the girl's screams lost a measure of intensity, became less shrill, and her struggles diminished. Neilson watched and waited, his hand poised on the syringe as the intravenous solution dripped steadily above the girl's head. At last she was spent, her desperate cries reduced to a hoarse moaning plea, her face slack, her limbs still, almost lifeless.

One by one, the exhausted nurses drifted away and busied themselves with other patients in the room. Dr.

Neilson pulled a stool near the head of the bed and sat, handing Jennifer the chart. He made a sign with his hand in the air for Jennifer to write. As he questioned the girl—Melanie, the chart said—Jennifer filled out the history form, her hand trembling slightly, her pulse beginning to slow. The first questions were routine. Name, Melanie Wardner. Age, twenty-five. Single. Shares an apartment with a secretary named Bea. A history of recurrent bladder infections. Dr. Bevins had treated her before, had said something about the tube which drained urine from her bladder being pinched. As Jennifer recorded answers to Neilson's questions, the angry flush of Melanie's cheeks gradually faded beneath her damp hair, and she clasped Dr. Neilson's hand in hers. When her voice slurred, Neilson softly repeated his question so Jennifer could hear. His voice was soothing, calm, and assured. Almost hypnotic. At length Melanie drifted off to sleep. Neilson folded her hand and placed it on the yellow blanket, carefully tucking the blanket edges beneath Melanie's arms as he stood. He took the chart from Jennifer as they approached the nurses' desk against the far wall. After writing several orders in the chart, he spoke briefly with the young head nurse and motioned for Jennifer to follow him out the door.

"That girl has an incredible tolerance for medication," he said as they approached the elevator. "And virtually no tolerance for pain."

"That was Stadol you gave her?"

He nodded. "Butorphanol tartrate. Eight milligrams intravenously." He waited for her reaction.

"Eight milligrams?"

"Exactly. Almost eight times the average dose. Follow her up closely, and see that she comes to the clinic when she's able. I want to determine her true pain threshold."

As the elevator arrived, Jennifer couldn't help commenting on the scene she had witnessed. "You were very kind to her."

Neilson narrowed his eyes slightly. "She was in pain." And he pressed the elevator button for the first floor.

In the animal laboratory that afternoon, Jennifer watched as Dr. Neilson tested and recorded pain responses and medications on guinea pigs and white rats. He explained as he worked, and said the experiments would be a significant part of Jennifer's duties. Nurse Kane had already applied tiny wires to the ears and feet of the guinea pigs. Jennifer cringed as Neilson pressed the control button that sent a painful stimulus to one fat and fuzzy little animal. Its squeaks and writhings made her withdraw instantly, and her concern must have shown on her face. She couldn't help but think of the little hamsters she had for pets as a child.

"It's a small stimulus," Neilson said. "They can't tell us how much it hurts, so we watch their brain waves and their vital signs."

Jennifer looked where he indicated, at the electroencephalographic recording, the little animal's brain waves squiggling across the lighted screen. A digital readout indicated the animal's pulse rate and blood pressure. A double fountain-pen-like needle rose and fell slowly on a revolving graph paper which Jennifer didn't understand.

"That records both temperature and perspiration. Some animals don't perspire like humans. When they do, it's a measure of stress, their reaction to the pain. Body temperature is another way to measure it, within limits."

Neilson increased the stimulus to level 6, and Jennifer watched the fuzzy animal's pulse rate and blood pressure jump and its temperature slowly rise. She felt herself wince when it began to squirm and shriek, but Neilson immediately stopped the stimulus. He picked up a loaded syringe with attached tiny needle and injected a clear liquid into the guinea pig's abdomen. The animal didn't appear to feel the injection. Jennifer did. Moments later, Neilson turned the pain stimulus dial up to 8 and pressed the button. Jennifer waited apprehensively for the little guinea pig's reaction. There was none. Pulse slow and steady. Blood pressure stable. Neilson turned the dial to 10. Same lack of reaction. Then 12. Nothing. At 18 on the dial, Jennifer caught herself leaning forward to see if the wires had somehow become detached. They were intact.

Jennifer had to consciously close her mouth when Neilson swung around on his stool to face her, smiling, his eyes questioning.

"I can't believe it," she said. "He doesn't feel a thing."

Neilson turned off the machine and stood. He walked to a metal cage across the small room and sat, flipping on the switch of a similar control panel. Inside the cage, a frisky white rat moved its head back and forth suspiciously, its whiskers testing the air. "The floor of the cage is wired," Neilson explained. "That little lever at the end dispenses a controlled dose of medication. The rat has learned to press the lever whenever he feels pain. Watch."

Jennifer instinctively half-turned away from the cage at the thought of hurting the animal, but forced herself to watch. Neilson had, after all, stopped the guinea pig's pain. He turned the dial to 6 and gave a short burst of pain stimulus to the floor of the cage. The white rat jumped straight up in the air, then scurried across the cage and pressed the plastic lever with his nose. A small amount of clear liquid squirted into a tiny glass container, like a watering trough, beside the lever. The rat lapped it up instantly, then sat on its haunches studying them, as if for praise. Neilson waited for several minutes, made some notes in an open notebook, then turned the dial to 8. The rat licked at his whiskers. He advanced the dial to 10. Finally, at 12, the rat calmly walked across the cage, pressed the lever, and lapped up the newly delivered liquid. Neilson turned off the machine.

"What's in the medication?" Jennifer asked.

"I don't know."

She wasn't sure she'd heard him right.

"The medicines are changed arbitrarily. It's a double-blind study, so to speak. We programmed a computer to select certain medications for each experiment. There's morphine, Demerol, codeine, Stadol, aspirin, heroin, and even an extract of marijuana. Also a couple of new drugs I've developed. I can't be objective about the results if I know which medication is being given. This way, I only record the effectiveness of each dose given. When the study is over, we'll see how the different drugs compare."

Jennifer nodded, then shook her head. "But somebody must know. Who fills the medicine vials or the rat's supply?"

"Nurse Kane and Josef. Josef attends the animals. But they only use what the computer has instructed. It's different each day."

"Is it the same with the patients? You don't know what you're giving them?"

Neilson took her arm and walked toward the door to the hall. "For the patients in the study, I don't know which medicine they receive. But some of the patients we see aren't in the study. Like the girl in recovery room. I'd love to have her in the study. With such a low pain threshold, she'd be ideal. But I couldn't let her hurt that badly. Maybe when she's recovered enough."

Nurse Kane was waiting at the reception desk when they came out of the lab. Two patients were seated on the long wooden benches in front of her. Without speaking, Kane directed the patients into the examining rooms, and handed a chart to Jennifer. Dr. Neilson entered the first exam room. Jennifer went into the second.

The young woman seated on Jennifer's examination table tried to smile but didn't quite make it. Her arms were folded across her abdomen, hunching her over slightly. The chart said number 1029. Jennifer extended her hand and introduced herself.

"I'm Lisa Waters," the waifish girl said. Short blond hair gave a pixie quality to her face, but the face should have been laughing or singing, with her little turned-up nose bouncing through the air as she danced, like the white ball in the movies that shows you which words to sing. Two tiny slash lines wrinkled her brow when she spoke. "I hurt so bad. Can you help me?"

3

Jennifer asked all the questions on the history form, and Lisa Waters answered eagerly. "It's the cramps. Every month the same thing. I can't work, do anything. I'm usually in bed two, three days."

Jennifer found it hard to believe the pain could be quite so bad; she'd learned to live with her own monthly discomfort. But she listened sympathetically.

"I've been fired from two jobs. They can't understand missing two or three days every month. And I have to work."

Jennifer noted on the history form that Lisa had lived alone since her parents were killed. She apparently supported herself as a secretary. "Have you taken anything for the pain?"

Lisa sighed. "Everything. Aspirin, Darvon. Maxigesic, Percodan. I even tried hypnosis. I still have to go to bed." She hunched forward again abruptly, as though trying to press her arms inside her abdomen. "I'm sorry," she said, chewing at a corner of her lip. "I know I sound silly. But it hurts."

Jennifer stood. "Pain is not silly, Lisa. Nobody likes to hurt. I want to do some tests on you. We need to find out how strong your pain is so we know how to treat it. Okay?"

There was a moment's hesitation. "Will the tests hurt?"

"Not any more than the pain you have now."

Lisa's big blue eyes darted toward the door, then back at Jennifer. "Okay. I guess."

Nurse Kane agreed to administer the pain-threshold tests with Jennifer watching. Lisa's hands shook slightly as the colored wires were attached to her temples and fingertips. Kane had to wipe Lisa's fingers dry twice before the adhesive would stick. Lisa looked up at Jennifer for reassurance. Jennifer smiled and nodded.

"Tell me when you feel the first sensation." Nurse Kane turned the dial from 0 to 1.

"I feel it," Lisa blurted out.

Kane narrowed her eyes, made a note on Lisa's chart. She turned the dial to number 2.

"Ouch, that stings," Lisa said, drawing her hands back from the table.

"Please don't jump or pull away," Nurse Kane said.

Lisa looked questioningly at Jennifer again, but put her hands back on the table. Kane raised the intensity level to 3. Beads of perspiration appeared on Lisa's upper lip. Kane waited for several seconds, then pressed the button.

"Oh, ouch, stop." Lisa jerked away so violently she stripped the adhesive pads from her fingertips, and the wires fell to the floor.

Nurse Kane flicked off the machine instantly and glared at Lisa. "You're being ridiculous. I told you to not pull away."

"It hurt," Lisa whimpered.

"The most you could have felt was a tiny shock," Kane countered.

Jennifer interrupted. "Lisa, we're only trying to help you. Nurse Kane is very busy, so you mustn't take up her time for nothing. If I perform the tests, and I promise to go real slow, will you try again? I need to learn."

Nurse Kane shifted her glare from Lisa to Jennifer. Jennifer ignored it, and smiled at Lisa. Finally Lisa nodded her head and bent to pick the fallen wires from the floor.

Dr. Neilson came out of the examining room at that moment, said good-bye to his patient, and walked over to where they sat. "Mind if I watch?"

Nurse Kane stood abruptly and marched out toward the reception desk. Jennifer nervously wiped Lisa's moist fingers again and applied the adhesive pads and wires. She tried to remember exactly which dial did what. Neilson's staring over her shoulder didn't help. She turned the dial back to zero and switched on the machine. On an impulse, she removed one of the wires from Lisa's fingertips and applied it to one of her own. Neilson didn't comment, but Lisa's widened eyes followed her every move.

Very slowly Jennifer got Lisa up to a level of 3 on the dial before Lisa asked her to stop.

"Is that about the same pain intensity you feel from your cramps, Lisa?"

She nodded. "Almost. But it's different."

Jennifer switched off the machine and turned to face Dr. Neilson. "Shall I give her a prescription?"

Neilson stood. "I think she'd be perfect for the study. I'll ask Nurse Kane to give her something." He asked Lisa, "Can you come in regularly for the next few weeks?"

She wiped at the adhesive on her fingers where the wires had been. "If it will help. I'm not working just now."

Neilson nodded and went out toward Kane's desk. Lisa lightly touched Jennifer's arm as she began to rise. "Dr. Barton, did that hurt you as much as it did me?"

Jennifer saw the concern in Lisa's eyes. She couldn't admit she'd hardly felt it. "It hurt, Lisa. Maybe not the same, but it hurt."

As Nurse Kane attended to Lisa's medications, Dr. Neilson halted Jennifer in the hall. "That was very nicely handled, doctor."

She felt herself start to flush. "Thank you."

He glanced at his watch. "It's almost five o'clock. May I buy you a drink?"

His question was so abrupt it caught her off balance. She started to accept his offer, but gave it a second thought. "Thank you, but I must do some grocery shopping before the stores close. I'm almost out of everything."

He squeezed her arm. "Another time."

Jennifer nodded, and went to collect her purse and sweater. As she pulled open the door to the back room where Nurse Kane had instructed her to leave her personal things, she almost yelped, coming face to chest with an enormous and unkempt man who charged right into her, almost toppling her backward. He grunted as he caught himself on the doorframe and stared dully down at her, his breath foul. His long face was slack, his mouth open and unmoving, as though ready to drool spittle down his chin, his features coarse.

"What do you want?" she demanded.

He blinked slowly and held a trash basket toward her, as though offering it in apology. "I'm Josef," he said in a basso-profundo voice. "Who are you?"

Jennifer's heart pounded in her ears as Dr. Neilson interrupted her anguish. "I see you've met Josef, Dr. Barton. Josef, this is our new associate."

Josef nodded; then a slow grin opened his face like a fault line.

"I'm through in the lab for the day, Josef," Neilson said. "Nurse Kane will tell you what to prepare for tomorrow."

The man nodded his enormous head, still grinning at Jennifer. "Yes, doctor," he said, and lumbered past them into the hall.

"Don't let Josef upset you," Neilson said, touching her arm. "He's much brighter than he appears. And a damn good worker."

After Jennifer left the clinic, she stopped by the university library. She wanted to read up on the physiology of pain and on the properties of currently available pain medications. She flipped through the card catalog under "Analgesics" and asked the computer operator to do a search for any articles by Dr. Franklyn Neilson. To her surprise, there were more than thirty articles by Neilson in the world literature. Twelve of the articles were in journals in the stacks of the library. Instead of going grocery shopping, Jennifer took his articles home to read.

When she opened the door to her small efficiency apartment, she almost stepped on an envelope beneath the door. She dropped her purse on the sofa and opened the envelope to discover her rent was due. Damn. The seven hundred dollars she had to her name would barely cover the amount due. And she wouldn't get paid from the pain clinic till the end of the month. She dropped the notice on the cushion beside her and slowly unbuttoned her sweater. She'd speak with the super in the morning. Maybe he'd let her pay half now, the rest on the first of February. At least that would leave her some money for food.

Jennifer nibbled at a turkey TV dinner and was fascinated with the fourth of Neilson's pain articles when the phone jangled through her concentration at eight-thirty that evening.

"He's a terminal-cancer patient," the nurse said. "Dr. Warren wants a consult on his pain medication tonight."

Fifteen minutes later, Jennifer had made the long trek through the tunnel under a drenched First Avenue, and took the elevator to the fifth floor of the enormous hospital. On the Head and Neck Ward, she was directed to bed fourteen by the evening nurse, an indifferent girl.

"Mr. Jackson?" Jennifer asked.

The thin white-haired man strained to open his cadaveric eyes, and tried to focus on Jennifer. His pupils were no larger than pinholes. She could have made the diagnosis of tongue cancer from across the room. Bulging lumps on both sides of his neck signaled rampant spread of the malignancy into his cervical lymph nodes. Reddened, irritated skin outlined by purple marking-pen lines from behind his ears almost to his collarbones and across the midline of his neck were evidence of the massive doses of radiation therapy the old man had received. Pain showed in his lined face and clouded his sunken eyes. He slowly lifted a bony hand, clawlike, and accepted Jennifer's handshake.

She introduced herself and asked the questions necessary to complete her questionnaire. A review of Walter Jackson's chart confirmed her suspicions of the diagnosis—carcinoma of the base of his tongue—and of his treatment by cobalt irradiation. He had smoked two packs of cigarettes daily for forty-five of his sixty years, and admitted to drinking two pints of whiskey per day. Jennifer mentally doubled that amount when she examined him and felt his firm liver edge eight centimeters below his scrawny rib cage. When she completed her examination, she hesitated to order any stronger pain medications on her own. Jackson was currently receiving a hundred milligrams of Demerol every three hours, was probably already addicted to the drug, and swore it gave him no relief from his suffering.

"I haven't slept a wink in four days," he said, his sallow cheeks tight as a death mask against the outlines of his skull. His watery eyes almost twinkled for an instant. "I'm not afraid of dying, doctor. But I can't go on suffering this way."

Jennifer excused herself, went to the telephone at the nurses' station, and asked for Dr. Neilson's home number. He wasn't in. In desperation she called and asked the nursing supervisor for Nurse Kane's number, and reached her on the first try. She explained Walter Jackson's diagnosis and situation. "He probably can't live for more than a few weeks," Jennifer said. "And he's in excruciating pain. I'd like to discuss him with Dr. Neilson."

"Record your findings in his chart," Nurse Kane said. "I'll come over right away and start him on treatment."

"I'll be glad to write the orders," Jennifer said.

"I'm authorized to medicate patients on Dr. Neilson's orders. There's no need for you to stay." And she hung up.

Jennifer informed Walter Jackson of Nurse Kane's

imminent visit with new medication, talked with him about the Yankees and the old Dodgers, and went home. She almost turned around to go back when she got off the creaky elevator in Brigton House, to offer him the sympathy and compassion she knew Nurse Kane wouldn't provide, but decided what he really wanted was relief from his pain.

At home, Jennifer withdrew a third of the water from her goldfish bowl and added clean water. She lowered her face to the side of the bowl, where her two little friends watched and waited. "You're very lucky little fish," she said. "You've got each other. And I love you." Though she knew she shouldn't, she dropped a single pellet into the bowl for Sushi, and crushed another for Saki. "A little special treat," she said.

Later, frustrated and depressed over Mr. Jackson, Jennifer changed into her yellow terry-cloth robe and curled on a corner of the sofa to read.

By ten-thirty, Walter Jackson had been transferred to one of the beds reserved for Dr. Neilson's patients on the second floor. Nurse Kane assigned him number 1032 and administered an injection with the same code number. At eleven P.M. Walter Jackson was fast asleep, a hint of a smile visible on his sunken lips above an incongruously bloated, lumpy neck.

After finally convincing her building superintendent to accept half her rent now and the rest later, Jennifer arrived at the Pain Control Clinic at eight-fifteen Tuesday morning, and saw an unending stream of patients until after eleven. She was amazed at the accuracy of Neilson's pain measurements from one of the articles she had read the evening before. She tested patients with migraine headaches, ranging from 12 to 18 on the pain-threshold scale, a man with a tooth abscess at 18, and a laborer with low-back pain at 6, though he said it often got worse. Jennifer was delighted to see Lisa Waters, smiling and happy, just before noon.

"You guys are fantastic," Lisa said. "I don't feel a thing."

"Your cramps are gone?" Jennifer asked.

"No, but they don't hurt. I mean, I still feel the spasms, but there's no pain."

Lisa readily agreed to undergo the pain-threshold testing, and Jennifer was amazed at her findings. At a dial setting of 12, Lisa merely smiled and wrinkled her pixie nose with delight, while the day before she had pulled away in agony at a setting of 3. Jennifer curiously attached one of the wires to her own finger again, and repeated the testing at a setting of 12. She almost jumped off her seat when a searing pain shot through her finger and up her arm, causing her to yank her finger free of the wire. Lisa smothered a giggle with one hand while Jennifer fought to regain her self-control.

"I'm sorry for laughing," Lisa said. "But I just feel so good. It's like some kind of high to not feel any pain."

Nurse Kane interrupted before Jennifer could comment. "Dr. Neilson wants you in the animal lab this afternoon, doctor. I'll finish up here."

Jennifer couldn't be sure whether the heat in her cheeks was from her anger and shock of the pain she had felt or from her instinctive dislike of Nurse Kane. She forced herself to rise, and turned to Lisa Waters. "I'm glad you're feeling better, Lisa. See you Thursday."

Lisa nodded. "I'll be here. And thank you, Dr. Barton."

Jennifer decided to visit Walter Jackson before she went to lunch. She collected the African-violet plant she had decided to give him, and went to the Head and Neck Ward on the fifth floor.

"He's been transferred to two," a nurses' aide told her. "Room 214."

On the second floor, Jennifer was confused by the information she received.

"Discharged this morning. First thing."

"But he's dying," Jennifer protested. "In severe pain."

The fat floor nurse shrugged. "He looked fine to me. Walked out of here like a sixteen-year-old."

"Who wrote the order for his discharge?"

"The signature said Dr. Neilson. If you're unhappy, talk to him. I don't make the rules."

Jennifer shook her head, put the African violet back in the storage room, then went to lunch.

While Jennifer stood in the snaillike cafeteria line, Lisa Waters grinned as Nurse Kane raised the dial of the pain machine to 16 and pressed the control button.

"It feels good," Lisa said. "It tingles." She giggled.

Nurse Kane switched off the machine and stood. "I'll be right back. I have an injection for you."

"Can't I have the medicine I had yesterday? The one I drank?"

Kane didn't answer, but returned seconds later with a filled hypodermic syringe. Lisa reluctantly rolled up her sweater sleeve, turned her head away, and screwed up her tiny face in anticipation before the needle pierced her vein. Her last comment before she lost consciousness was, "Hey . . . I didn't even feel it." Moments later, Josef carried Lisa Waters' limp form down the narrow corridor behind the clinic and placed her on a bed in a Spartan gray room after Nurse Kane unlocked the door. While Kane placed Lisa's purse and overcoat on the floor near the bed, Josef hissed under his breath and kicked, too late, at a scrawny brown rat which darted out from beneath Lisa's bed and scurried through the open door, its nails scratching and slipping on the dingy tiled floor.

4

After lunch, Jennifer accompanied Dr. Neilson to see Melanie Wardner on the fourteenth floor of the private wing of the hospital. Melanie was dozing when they entered, the only sound in her room a steady dripping of blood-tinged urine into a glass bottle tied to the frame of her bed. The bulkiness of the bandages on her abdomen was evident beneath the sheet which covered her. Melanie suddenly opened frightened eyes as Neilson studied her chart. "It's starting to wear off," she whined, fumbling for the nurse's call button at her side.

Neilson caught her hand and held it in both of his. "It's all right, Melanie. I'm Dr. Neilson. Try to describe what you feel."

Melanie shook her head. "It burns something terrible. And it aches, like somebody's jumped on my stomach and squashed it." A tear trickled down one pale temple.

"Have you ever had a pain anything like this?"

Melanie shook her head, chin trembling. "I had a bad ear infection once, when I was twelve. It was awful, but nothing like this."

Neilson nodded, and wiped a tear from her temple with his thumb. "The nurses tell me you required an injection every two hours all night. Do you think you can get by with a little less today?"

Melanie turned her head away for a moment, then looked up at Neilson, pleading with her eyes. "It hurts so bad, doctor. And he promised it wouldn't hurt."

"It isn't safe to take this much medication, Melanie. It can be habit-forming. Addicting."

The girl chewed at her lower lip and sniffed wetly. "Have you ever hurt this bad, doctor?" She turned her scrunched-up red eyes to Jennifer. Jennifer swallowed, waited for Neilson to break the silence.

"No," Neilson said. "But I've seen many people who have." After a long pause he continued. "Melanie, there's a new drug I'm working with. It doesn't appear to cause addiction. Would you like me to try it on you?"

She dabbed at one eye with the back of her free hand. "Will it stop the pain?"

Neilson hesitated. "I can't promise, but I believe it will."

Melanie sobbed once, then grabbed her abdomen as if afraid it might split open. She began to whine, squeezing her eyes tightly shut until her pale face flushed crimson. Finally she spoke, whispering. "I'll try anything, doctor. Anything."

Neilson took a folded sheet of paper from his white coat and asked Melanie to sign at the bottom of the printed page. She strained to scribble her signature, without reading the page. Neilson turned to Jennifer, asked her to sign as a witness. Jennifer quickly scanned the words, a consent form to permit Neilson to administer an experimental drug to Melanie. It essentially said that while the drug had been tested extensively in animals, its effectiveness and safety in humans had not been established.

When Jennifer signed and returned the form to Neilson, he took a vial of clear liquid from his pocket and poured about five cc's into a paper cup beside the anxious girl's bed, then handed it to her. Melanie accepted the cup, blinked long wet eyelashes twice, and drank it, returning her head to the pillow.

"It tastes like water," she said. "How long does it take to work?"

Neilson patted her hand. "Not long. Try to sleep now. I'll look in later."

In the hall outside, Jennifer asked about the drug.

"It's the work of a lifetime," Neilson said. "It's basically a neuropeptide, like those occurring naturally in the brain and adrenal glands. It seems to stimulate the body to form its own pain medication, an enkephalin-type substance."

"Like the endorphins?" Jennifer asked.

"Exactly. Pain, stress, exercise, sexual excitement, perhaps other stimuli, cause the brain to release endorphins, opiatelike substances. They're basically similar to morphine, as all our effective medications are. But they're natural, not synthetic, nature's own morphine. So it works without side effects."

The elevator arrived, interrupting Neilson. Jennifer asked what the drug was called.

"Chemically, it's a name about this long." He spread his hands far apart. "For now, I call it Opain."

"What's in it?"

Neilson tilted his head to one side, peering over his glasses at Jennifer. He smiled and touched her arm. "That, my dear pretty doctor, is top-secret."

Jennifer nodded her understanding, but felt a tinge of rejection at his mistrust. "Have you used it on people?"

His eyes flickered for an instant. "I'm sure I have."

"You don't know?"

He smiled. "The computer knows. It's part of the study."

"But what about Melanie? She's not part of the study."

The elevator landed on the first floor. "Maybe she will be," he said. "First, I want to know how she reacts."

Neilson excused himself and instructed Jennifer to go to the animal lab. "Dr. West can show you what to do."

As Jennifer walked toward the lab adjacent to the Pain Control Clinic, Laniet Teague mashed the control button in a nearby room, her cheeks as red as her sodden hair. She pressed her thumb harder and harder against the control, grunting with effort as the numbers on the readout slowly climbed past 26 and registered 27. Her breath came in short bursts as the pain tore through her fingers and toes and stabbed the raw nerve endings in her arms. The sensation beneath the cast on her fractured right arm was almost sexual, as though a hundred orgasms were encased in the plaster itself, crying out to be released. She moaned with the incredible stimulation, and hardly noticed the metallic taste of blood on her lower lip as she fought the cobwebs of darkness crowding the edges of her mind. Near-bursting blue veins strained against the delicate red skin of her forehead and neck as the number 28 glowed in the swirling distance. The high, keening sounds in her ears changed abruptly to a sharp cry of pain and ecstasy, vaguely like her own voice in the distance as the numbers advanced to 29 and all abruptly went black. Josef unfolded his arms from where he leaned against the back wall, and came to her side. He turned off the control-panel power, scrawled a notation in the open notebook beside Laniet's chair, and disconnected the wires from her temples, fingers, and toes. After securing the unconscious girl to her bed, Josef looked in on Lisa Waters in the adjacent room. He smiled and nodded to himself that Lisa remained asleep, ankles and wrists securely bound to the metal side rails of her bed.

Josef turned at the door and stopped to stare at the miniature sleeping girl, her full breasts rising and falling with each breath, straining the silken material of her blouse. A thick tongue slid across his heavy lips, and he walked to a cupboard against the near wall and took out a white hospital gown. By removing one limb restraint at a time, he gradually undressed Lisa, his fingers trembling slightly when he unsnapped the catch on her brassiere behind her back. He was careful to fold and stack her blouse, slacks, and underclothing on the shelf in the cupboard, turning to stare at her nakedness as he worked. He slipped her left arm through the sleeve of the hospital gown, and was about to untie her right arm again when she made a soft, cooing noise in her sleep, and strained to lift one knee against the restraints. Josef stiffened, waited. But Lisa only tossed her head to one side and resumed her rhythmic breathing. Her angulation raised her right breast, its pink nipple pointing straight at Josef's face, rising and falling like the swells in a deep sea. He carefully pulled the gown over her triangle of blond thatch, only slightly brushing his hand against her as he did. His Adam's apple worked as he spread his hand over her exposed breast and felt the rising prominence of her nipple meet his palm.

"Josef."

He turned instantly, recoiling from Lisa's breast as though stung by a wasp.

"I'll finish that." Nurse Kane's gaze fixed on his face.

"The other one passed out again," he said.

"Did you note the intensity?"

He nodded, backing away from the bed, but watching intently as Nurse Kane pulled the gown over Lisa's breast.

Kane ignored his leer. "Go to the lab, Josef. Play dumb and keep in the background. But let me know what Dr. West and Jennifer Barton discuss. I have the feeling young Dr. Barton may become a problem. Watch her."

By the time Jennifer reached the lab, David West had the animals prepared for the afternoon experiments, and seemed genuinely happy to see her. "Try not to knock any tables over today." He grinned.

"I'm surprised you didn't set one against the door," Jennifer answered. "As a booby trap."

West laughed, then turned to a pair of cages behind him. "You may not like this one, but it's a controlled experiment to determine pain tolerance."

Jennifer was almost certain from his tone she wouldn't like it. She took two tentative steps forward to look over his shoulder, hardly breathing. The musty rodent-stench of the lab stuck in her nostrils as she waited.

West lined up two identical cages, each housing a

frisky but curious white rat, and connected the input wires to the bottom of each cage.

"They're sisters," he said.

He turned the control dial up to 3, and pressed the button that gave a short burst of pain to the bottoms of their feet. Each rat squealed, turned quickly, and ran to the plastic lever at the end of its cage. Seconds later, each lapped at the liquid which squirted into its glass trough. West waited, making notations in a book. Josef entered the lab behind Jennifer, smiled briefly at her when she turned, and busied himself in a far corner, cleaning a cage.

West raised the intensity dial to 4, repeated the pain stimulus, and recorded identical reactions of the two rats. By the time he was up to 7, the white rat in the first cage sat majestically on her haunches and ignored the stimulus, while the second scurried about frantically, repeatedly pressing the lever and lapping up the liquid as though she had found a cool stream in the middle of a sun-baked desert. Jennifer recoiled with each stimulus, watching the second rat squirm and squeal, its pulse, blood pressure, and respiration climbing steadily.

"That's enough," she said, grasping West's shoulder.

He turned to face her. "Hey. It's not that bad."

She shook her head. "I don't like it. She's in pain."

West studied Jennifer for a moment. "From the look on your face, you'd think you were in the cage."

Jennifer shuddered. "Please. No more." She tried to smile.

David West shrugged his eyebrows. "I only follow Neilson's instructions. But I never take them above their viable tolerance level."

Jennifer didn't understand.

"When the heart rate and blood pressure rise above a tolerance level, they die. They quit drinking, and keel over."

Jennifer had to sit down. "From pain?"

West nodded. "I only saw it once. It was pretty bad."

"How could you?" she demanded.

He shook his dark head. "We didn't know. We had

one with a threshold so low it blew a cerebral artery at level five on the pain scale."

Jennifer felt a sudden chill in the room, hugged her arms to her body. "That's sick."

West frowned slightly, swallowed, then spoke. "It's called research. There was no way to know. And an innocent little rat died so that maybe someday people won't."

Jennifer decided against reacting to his defensive tone. She knew he was right—new drugs that might save millions of lives or relieve humans of their suffering had to be tested some way—but she didn't know if she'd be able to see it through. She had to try to understand pain. To learn how to control it. But she couldn't bear the idea of being the instrument which produced it—in animals or humans. She stood and walked across the lab, speaking before she turned. "Do you think Neilson's found the answer?"

West hesitated before answering. "I think he's the one who will."

She turned to look into his serious face. "Is he that good?"

West switched off the power console. "Did you know he developed Endolor?"

Jennifer searched her memory. The change of subject allowed her to partially regain her composure. "That's a Fost-Walker drug. Supposedly with no respiratory depression, right?"

West nodded. "Neilson worked for Fost-Walker. So did Nurse Kane. He developed the drug on his own time, but Fost-Walker won rights to the formula in a lawsuit."

"I hear it doesn't work so well."

West grinned. "Read the early reports on it. It was nearly perfect. Phenomenal pain relief with no sedation. Minimal addiction. It was to be the wonder drug of the century."

"So?"

"So, Fost-Walker sued Neilson and got the exclusive rights to it. They spent millions of dollars and eight years to get FDA approval. Neilson bankrupted in the court battles. But somehow the formula got changed when Neilson quit to come here."

Jennifer was shocked. "You think he changed it?"

West extended his arms, palms up. "What would you think? And you can't blame him. He did the research in his spare time. His own lab. I'd say he got even. It's what those men who developed the electrical painkiller machine should have done."

"Which machine?"

"A few years back, a couple of guys developed an electrical stimulator that interrupted painful sensations. Sort of the same principle as acupuncture. They sold out to a major drug company with the understanding they'd split any profits made off the machine."

"I haven't heard of it."

"Almost nobody has. The company never promoted the machine. They already had the largest over-the-counter pain medicine on the market. They killed the idea to protect their own product. So the inventors sued the company."

Jennifer couldn't believe it. "Are you sure?" she asked.

"They were awarded over a hundred and seventy million dollars when they went to court," West said. "That gives you an idea of what kind of profits there are in pain treatments."

Jennifer's thoughts were interrupted by a loud squeal and snapping noise behind her. When she turned, horrified, the white rat Neilson had used in the experiment the day before backed against the wire of one end of its cage, and suddenly lunged full speed at the far end, banging its head against the cage so hard the plastic lever snapped off and clattered to the floor near her feet. Blood dripped from the rat's nose as it lay stunned for a moment, then turned and raced to the opposite end, wedging its bloody whiskers and pointed nose into the tiny square openings of the wire cage as it struggled to its feet and reeled unsteadily around.

"Stop it," she cried, reaching for the door to the cage.

Before Jennifer could pry the door open, Josef appeared at her side and grabbed the cage from the table.

"It's okay, doctor," he said. "I'll take care of it." Josef turned quickly and unlocked a rear exit, carrying the frantic rat and cage into another room, slamming the door behind him.

Jennifer turned to West. "What was that all about? Yesterday that rat sat and ignored the pain stimuli. It must be a reaction to the medicine."

"Nobody knows what's in the medicine," West said, "except the computer. Write it down in the notebook. Neilson will figure it out."

Jennifer thought she'd explode. "Don't you even give a damn?"

West's face flushed. "Yes, I give a damn. But I'm not privy to what's in Neilson's computer."

"That animal had a very abnormal reaction. He could have killed himself. And you don't seem to care."

West slammed the notebook closed. "Look, doctor, I care. I care a hell of a lot. But I'm a scientist. I can't squeal and whimper every time somebody hurts. Somebody has to be objective."

"So you repress all emotion. Is that it?"

"No, I don't repress it. I just don't wear it on my sleeve." He looked as though he had something more to say, but didn't. He wheeled around to the lab notebook and opened it, making rapid notes, the back of his neck red with anger.

Jennifer stood stiffly silent for several moments, considering what he'd said. At least she'd gotten a reaction from him. Finally she asked, trying to keep her voice calm, "Have you seen reactions like that before?"

West busied himself with the next experiment. "No."

Something in his tone made Jennifer question his answer. But he quickly diverted her attention to the guinea pig in the cage beside him. She watched as he adjusted the dials, checked each connection. His fingers moved swiftly, his eyes absorbing every detail, his concentration total. As he worked, Jennifer felt her tension relax. He was very gentle with the little animal.

When he finally spoke, his voice was professional and in control. "This proves you can raise your pain threshold by repeated exposure," he said. He set the dial at pain level 7 and pressed the control button. The guinea pig stood staring at them curiously, then slowly paced the length of the cage, unconcerned. "Samson here went bonkers at level three only four weeks ago," he said. When West increased the pain to level 8, Samson hastened to the tiny trough and lapped away at the clear liquid.

West's concern with the experiment was so contagious that Jennifer became caught up in it, as though their heated discussion had never occurred.

"What's in the medicine?" she asked.

West switched off the apparatus and turned. "This one I do know. Water."

Jennifer was amazed. "Then why does he drink it?"

"He was conditioned with small amounts of Demerol. Now he drinks the water, and his pain threshold goes up. Like a placebo, a sugar pill."

"Only he doesn't know it's sugar-pill water, right?"

"People take sugar pills and get relief, we call it psychological. I suspect Samson disproves that. More likely, repeated exposure to mild pain stimulates the body's own morphine."

"The endorphins," Jennifer said.

West nodded. "And enkephalin. Do you remember how bad it hurt to step barefoot on a bee when you were little? Or get a shot?"

"Who could ever forget?"

"Why does pain seem so much stronger in a child?" he asked. "You have to learn the hard way what *hot* means. How pain feels. A sore throat. Earache. The colic. I believe it's a method of conditioning the endorphin-stimulating mechanism, so you don't feel as much pain when you're older. The more you hurt, the more natural morphine your brain squirts into your system's trough."

Jennifer turned to see Josef reenter the lab, but he ignored them, tending the animals.

West continued. "When they autopsy little Samson there, I predict he'll have two or three times the endorphins and enkephalin of a similar animal that hasn't been stimulated."

Jennifer had the feeling Samson's eyes suddenly dilated, then narrowed, as if he understood. "I hope they don't expect me to do the autopsy."

"Josef and Neilson do them. They send the critical organs to the path lab and biochemistry."

"And the bodies?"

"Cremate them." West lowered and quavered his voice, ghoul-like. "Neilson took over part of the old morgue. The crematorium."

"That isn't funny. I didn't know morgues had crematoriums."

"What do you think they do with the arms and legs they remove? Surgical specimens?"

Jennifer had never thought about it. It made sense. But she preferred to change the subject. "How many patients are in Neilson's study?"

West poured himself a cup of coffee, extending an empty cup to Jennifer, which she refused. "Over a thousand, I guess. We're up to code number 1057."

"Isn't that enough to stop and analyze the results?"

"Neilson wanted a thousand. But you know how patients are. Some don't come back for follow-up. Others move away. I'd say he's pretty close, but only the computer knows." He waved one hand in the air expansively.

Nurse Kane opened the hall door to the lab, her face impassive. "Dr. Barton, there's an emergency consult in obstetrics. Labor room. Dr. Neilson wants you to meet him there."

Jennifer hurried to the obstetrical floor after picking up a supply of history forms from the clinic. Neilson was already at the bedside of a shrieking, wailing, very pregnant small brown woman who writhed in her sweat-soaked bed. Jennifer was unable to record any information on her forms, and could hardly hear Neilson's questions for the woman's incessant cries, half in English, half in Spanish. Two angry nurses and a bearded black orderly pinned the woman's arms and legs while an O.B.

resident performed a rectal exam amid her hysterical screams.

"She's dilating," the resident said, stripping off his glove. "About another hour." To Neilson he said, "I'm afraid to give her anything more. Fetal heartbeat has slowed already. The baby wouldn't breathe for a week."

Neilson nodded, placed Maria Ortez's chart on the bedside table, and took the same glass container from his pocket that Jennifer had seen in Melanie Wardner's room. He poured a measure of the clear liquid into a cup and waited for a lull in Maria's struggles between labor pains. Without a word, he lifted her sweaty head from the pillow and held the cup to her lips. Her dark brown eyes opened wide, like a trapped animal's, but she gulped the liquid down, licking her lips afterward like a dehydrating fox. Seconds later, Neilson gave an injection in her exposed buttock, and they left.

Jennifer questioned his failure to have the consent form signed.

"Later," he said. "There's no way to make her understand now."

"Was that Opain?"

He nodded.

"The injection or the oral liquid?"

Neilson stared down at her. "Both."

As they neared the end of the hall, Neilson turned to look at two nurses in short blue uniforms pushing a bed hurriedly past. On the bed was a howling, straining, red-faced woman whose abdomen mounded up like a camel's hump. "Looks like twins," Jennifer said.

"At least."

At the elevator, Jennifer asked, "Have you used Opain on pregnant women?"

"The injection. The oral preparation's new."

She hesitated, but asked, "It doesn't depress fetal respiration? Affect the baby?" She slid into the crowded elevator beside Neilson, one breast almost crushed against his arm.

He didn't answer until they emerged on the first floor. "Opain is the perfect painkiller." His eyes were level, intense, fixed on her face, but his voice was warm, understanding. "There is no respiratory depression. In the mother or the baby. I've used it in thousands of animals."

Jennifer swallowed hard. Though his tone was friendly, his stare was challenging. "And in how many humans? Or does only the computer really know?"

Neilson stood unblinking for several moments. "Nine hundred and seventy-six before Maria Ortez. Enough for me to know it's what I've dreamed of all my life. Not enough for the FDA to allow its release."

Before Jennifer could respond, Neilson wheeled and walked away, his white coat billowing out behind him like a new sail in the first puff of a freshening breeze.

Somebody tapped Jennifer's shoulder as she watched Neilson round the corner, causing her to almost jump, startled.

"You're from the pain clinic?" the puffy-eyed woman asked.

Jennifer said she was.

"Please help me find my daughter. She still hasn't come home."

Jennifer remembered when she smelled the cheap wine on the woman's breath and saw how she held the crumpled handkerchief to one side of her mouth as she spoke. She couldn't recall the name.

"Laniet Teague. Red hair, like mine. But pretty. Has a cast on one arm."

5

———••⬧⬧⬧••———

Jennifer was surprised not to see Nurse Kane at the reception desk in the Pain Control Clinic. Mrs. Teague stood nervously in front of the counter-type desk, a wisp of red hair peeking out from under her faded purple scarf, one liver-spotted hand grasping the counter's edge while Jennifer searched for the appointment books. At last she found three large books in an unlocked drawer on the bottom shelf and extracted the one covering current appointments. She ran her finger down the columns of names and numbers. No Laniet Teague.

"Is there anything about a nine-nine-something?" the woman asked,

Jennifer asked her to repeat.

"She said they called her nine-nine-something. I'm not good at numbers. Never was. Maybe a six. Or seven." She coughed into her handkerchief.

Jennifer studied the alcoholic woman's ectropic eyes, then flipped back to the first page of December appointments, reading the code numbers. She found 995, Robert Brown; 998, Felicia Washington. Number 996 was on the fourth of December, Johnny Rodriguez. She was up to December 23 when Nurse Kane slammed the appointment book closed, almost on Jennifer's fingers.

"Who gave you permission to remove my records?" Kane demanded.

Jennifer felt the heat burn its way out of her collar and up her neck. She heard her own voice shake when she spoke, meeting Kane's glare. "I'm trying to help this woman."

Mrs. Teague muffled a wheezing cough.

"I told her there's no Laniet Teague in our clinic," Kane said as though the woman didn't exist. She replaced the heavy appointment book on the bottom shelf and locked the drawer. "Is there anything else?" she asked Mrs. Teague.

The woman's eyes went dull, hopeless. Her shoulders drooped. "I just hope Laniet's not on that dope again. She was doing so good." Mrs. Teague started to leave, but turned to Jennifer. "Thank you anyway, doctor." Jennifer took the woman's phone number, said she'd call if Laniet came by.

Nurse Kane quickly brushed past Jennifer, as though to leave.

"Just a minute," Jennifer said.

Kane turned around, her tinted blond head cocked slightly to one side, her expression almost amused. For the first time, Jennifer noticed the tiny scar running vertically just in front of Kane's ear. A face-lift scar. Jennifer mentally added ten years to Kane's apparent forty years, but it was of little concern at the moment.

"Why is there no number nine-ninety-seven in the records?" Jennifer asked.

"That's hardly your concern."

Jennifer forced herself to sound calm. "I merely asked a question. I work here too."

Kane's eyes went hard. "There are many numbers not in the book, doctor." Her tone was condescending. "Patients who don't show up for appointments. Ones who refuse treatment. Unless you have a better system, I suggest you concentrate on your patients and leave the record-keeping to me." She blinked once, turned to lock the clinic door, and marched off down the empty hall.

Jennifer walked toward the animal lab, but found the

door locked. There was no answer to her knock. Damn. She'd left her purse and sweater inside. She quickly searched her pockets, found the spare key to her apartment door. Angry with both herself and Nurse Kane, she took the elevator to the fourteenth floor to check on Melanie Wardner, curious to see if she had any less pain from her ruptured-bladder operation after taking Opain.

To Jennifer's surprise, Melanie was propped up in her hospital bed eating something the consistency of yogurt, but yellow. Jennifer introduced herself.

"Sure. With Dr. Neilson," Melanie said.

"Looks like you're feeling better."

"It's magic. Hardly hurts at all. Unless I cough."

Jennifer tried to make small talk about the weather and hospital food.

"You know, I was really mad when I woke up this way." Melanie indicated the clear drainage tube extending from under the covers to the urine bottle. "Dr. Bevins had told me it was nothing to dilate my pee tube."

Jennifer nodded her understanding.

"But he explained what happened. I was still mad at first, mostly from the pain. Now it doesn't hurt so bad, I know it wasn't really his fault. You know?"

Jennifer nodded again.

Melanie shrugged and smiled. "I guess these things just happen. But what lousy timing. I've got a million things I should be doing." She shook her head. "Anyhow, he says I'll be up and around in no time. Maybe go home by the weekend. He was by a few minutes ago."

Jennifer said she was delighted Melanie felt so much better, excused herself, and left, amazed. She had never seen anybody look that comfortable after abdominal surgery, let alone somebody with absolutely no pain tolerance, as Melanie had been the day before. She rode the elevator down to the obstetrical floor.

The O.B. charge nurse said Maria Ortez was in room 515, bed 3. She'd had a seven-pound baby boy. Both fine. Jennifer entered the four-bedded room and found Maria sleeping while the other three patients stopped their conversation and watched curiously. One smiled. Their flat abdomens told Jennifer they had already delivered. As she approached bed 3, Maria opened her eyes and pressed the bed control to raise her head and shoulders. Jennifer told her who she was.

Maria answered with a heavy Spanish accent. "I don' remember too good, doctor. But I know it don' hurt no more. Not so bad after I drink the medicine. You see my baby?"

Jennifer said she hadn't. But she promised to go by the nursery on her way out.

"Es a beautiful boy. My son. He gonna be big and strong, not like me. Not afraid. I feed him good." Maria touched her prominent breasts, bulging with milk under her thin gown.

Jennifer made a note in Maria's chart and walked to the nursery. After checking at the nurses' desk, she peered through the large glass window at the bassinets until one of the masked nurses held Juan Ortez up for display. He was dark brown, wrinkled, and thrashed one tiny fist from beneath the blue blanket, trying to find his open but soundless mouth. A healthy, bouncing baby boy. Jennifer was saddened to have noticed on the chart that Maria was unmarried. And the nurse had said no father had come to visit. Nobody to share Maria's proud moment, or to point theatrically through the plate-glass window and brag that Juan Belmondo Ortez had arrived to change the world. "Good luck, Juan," she said, waved a half-wave, and walked away.

On an impulse, Jennifer walked to the sixth floor and down a long hall to the plastic-surgery offices. Unfamiliar white-uniformed residents and interns passed hurriedly in the opposite direction, a few giving her the once-over from toe to head. She didn't feel very desirable in her white hospital skirt, blouse, and jacket, and ignored their appraisals. She did pull her jacket closed over her full breasts, however.

The secretary in the chief of Plastic Surgery's office said Dr. Bronson had finished his appointments, and showed Jennifer inside.

Bronson didn't rise from his seat behind an expansive

mahogany desk, but leaned back in his leather chair and greeted Jennifer warmly. He was her image of the ideal plastic surgeon, immaculate and silver-haired, tan even in January, with blue eyes that seemed to catch whatever light was in the room and reflect it. "How are things in Pain Control? I hope you haven't forgotten how to operate." He indicated the seat in front of his desk, a Louis XIV, she thought.

Jennifer sat, exchanged brief pleasantries, then asked about her fellowship.

Bronson furrowed his elegant brow. "I'm sure we'll get funding by March or April. You just hang in there."

Jennifer assured him she would.

"When are you supposed to start in Atlanta?" he asked.

"July. But I think they'll wait a couple of months. I want to finish the full fellowship."

Bronson nodded confidently. "For somebody as bright and pretty as you, I'm sure they will." He shook his head. "I often long for the days before the government got involved in hospital finances. When we could plan our staffing requirements and stick to them."

Jennifer said she understood. "I just wanted to thank you for getting the job for me," she said. "To tide me over."

Bronson stood, walked her to the door with one arm around her shoulder. "It's the least I could do. I'm glad I could help out. I'm doing a face lift and breast reduction tomorrow morning. You're welcome to come watch."

She thanked him and left, cramming herself into a packed but silent elevator to ride to the first floor. She stopped at the hospital entrance facing First Avenue and looked out through the glass doors. She had hoped to walk home outdoors, but a sleeting rain continued to fall outside. As much as she craved a breath of fresh air, she took the stairwell down toward the underground tunnel, acutely aware that it had been three days since she was outside.

Concentrating on the first steps of the concrete stairwell, Jennifer almost jumped when a bass voice spoke to her.

"Good night, Dr. Barton."

She felt her muscles tense when Josef grinned at her. He should get his teeth cleaned. He scuffed up the stairs toward her, a tray of food carefully balanced in his hands, still wearing his drab green workshirt and trousers and stained shoes.

"Josef," she said, forcing a half-smile.

"Mind opening the door for me?"

She hesitated, then walked back up to the landing and pulled open the door. His tray was loaded with cafeteria food. At least his hands looked clean, she thought. That's something. "You must be hungry," she said, standing well out of his path beside the door.

He grinned again and nodded. "Yes, ma'am. Thank you."

When the door closed behind his enormous back, Jennifer gave a little shiver and raced down toward the tunnel. She had considered asking Josef to unlock the lab door so she could retrieve her purse and sweater, but decided it wasn't worth it. She felt silly admitting it, but he gave her the creeps.

Ten minutes later, as Jennifer reached to put the key in the lock of her apartment door, she heard a scraping sound from inside, and her hand froze in midair. She held her breath and listened, her heart suddenly racing. Something moved beyond the door, like muffled footsteps, then a creaking sound. She turned quickly to look behind her, but the hallway was empty, the elevator door closed. Papers rustled from within. Josef's coarse, grinning face flashed before her eyes, leering at her. She started to call out, to demand to know who had invaded her home. The six-P.M. light from the hall window was gray and dim, casting no shadow around her, the single hallway bulb unlit.

In desperation, Jennifer tiptoed down the hall to the adjacent apartment, where she'd heard a man's voice two nights before, through the thin walls. She knocked softly at the door. No response. She hurried across the hall and knocked again, impatient and frightened.

"Who is it?" a woman's voice asked through the closed door.

"Neighbor," she whispered. She had to repeat it, louder.

The door barely opened on its chain, and a thin pale face peered out through the crack with one green eye.

"There's somebody in my apartment," Jennifer whispered. "Let me in."

The green eye widened. "A burglar?"

"I don't know. Please let me in. Call the police."

"My husband isn't home," the pale face said. "Call the super." She closed the door in Jennifer's face, slid home the bolt.

Jennifer wanted to pound on the door. To scream out at the woman's inhumanity. Instead, she hurried down the hall to the stairwell, careful to keep her heels from clacking against the wood floor. Downstairs, the stocky building superintendent irritably answered his door in undershirt and khaki trousers, chewing something. He held a can of beer in one hand. Jennifer had to wait while he put on his shoes, his round-faced wife giving her one annoyed glance from the flowered sofa in front of the television. Jennifer told him what she'd heard as they waited for the slow elevator.

Outside her apartment door they listened. No sound came from within. "Stand back," the super said, placing his key in the lock. "I used to be a security guard."

"What the hell do you want?" somebody inside demanded as the door swung open.

The super recoiled, then growled, "What are you doing here?"

Jennifer stepped forward to look inside. David West sat in her chair, his feet on her desk, a glass of wine in one hand and sheets of paper in the other. She quickly apologized to the superintendent, who stalked away shaking his balding head.

Jennifer slammed the door behind her, hands on hips, embarrassed and furious. "How did you get in and what are you doing in my apartment?"

West shrugged, his white teeth flashing against his olive skin. "You're welcome," he said, lifting her purse and sweater off the desk beside his feet.

She didn't move. "The door was locked."

He took a sip of wine. "No it wasn't. And you should buy better wine. This is terrible Chablis."

Jennifer's fright began to subside, but her pulse bounded in her ears as she advanced toward him. "How dare you invade my privacy. Just who do you think you are?" She swept his feet off the desk with one rapid movement.

West stood, arms in the air as if surrendering, and smiled. "Hey. White-flag time. I was only trying to do a favor."

Jennifer glanced back at her purse and sweater on the desk. Too annoyed to speak, she grabbed them up and hung them on the stand beside the door. When she turned, West stood with hands extended, brows raised in the universal questioning gesture.

"Well?" he asked. "Do I finish my wine?"

She exhaled an abrupt sigh. "How did you know where I live?"

"You said Brigton House. Your name's on the mailbox downstairs. Three-C."

She reluctantly gave in to his boyish grin. "Oh, what the hell," she said. "Sit down while I change."

After exchanging her white uniform for jeans and a cotton shirt, Jennifer emerged from the bathroom to find West sitting on the sofa. She opened a bottle of Moselle and joined him, even thanked him for bringing her things from the lab. After a glass each of the wine, they got around to shop talk.

"Have you ever had a patient disappear from the clinic?" she asked abruptly.

"All the time."

"I mean really disappear. No trace of them."

West set his wineglass on the table, turned to face her on the sofa, asked what she meant. She told him about Laniet Teague's mother, and the number, 997.

"Lots of patients don't keep appointments," he said. "They feel better, so they stop coming in."

Jennifer studied her hands. "I think Nurse Kane is lying."

"Whatever for? You said the mother is an alcoholic and the girl's been on drugs. They're not exactly models of stable personalities. The girl probably ran off."

Jennifer had to admit he could be right. But something in that mother's puffy eyes made her want to believe her. She was convinced that Laniet Teague, number 997, had been a patient at the Pain Control Clinic. And Kane had lied about it. Jennifer changed the subject and told him about Maria Ortez and her new baby, Juan. "That Opain really works."

"I've seen it," West said. "Neilson and Kane won't admit which drug is which, but it's easy to spot the patients on Opain injections. They just quit hurting."

"By mouth, too," Jennifer said.

"It only comes as an injection."

Jennifer told him about Melanie Wardner and Maria. How Neilson had them drink Opain.

West brushed a strand of long brown hair off Jennifer's cheek. "Must be new. I haven't used it."

Jennifer recognized the hungry look in West's dark eyes before she felt his hand gently slide down her neck. His gaze fell to her lips as he pulled her head to him. She was taken by surprise, both at the abruptness of his actions and at her lack of desire to resist. His mouth was soft and searching, and she felt her lips part of their own volition as his tongue probed and darted and teased. The sudden force of her own hungers frightened her, and she pulled away. "No," she said.

West leveled his gaze to hers, his eyes humid but flashing. "Now who's repressing their feelings?"

Jennifer retrieved her wine and sat back, shaken. "You are very unpredictable, Dr. West."

"You seemed to like it."

She turned to look at him. "Yes, I liked it. But I don't know if I like you."

Something flickered in his eyes. "Are you always that blunt?"

"I try to be honest," she said, sensing his hurt. "I don't dislike you, either. It's just a little sudden."

He seemed to accept her statement, but toyed with his wineglass before speaking. "See what happens when I show my feelings?"

She couldn't help herself. "Don't tell me I'm your first rejection experience."

West took a deep breath, but smiled. "No. I've had my share." His expression made her regret her words immediately, though she doubted if many girls had ever turned him down.

"I'm sorry, David. It isn't you. It's me."

"Sure." He finished his wine. "Look, I really came by to apologize for blowing off at you in the lab today."

"I asked for it."

He didn't seem to hear. "I don't like losing control. You're new here, and a little uptight. That's normal. I guess I haven't helped much."

She touched his arm. "You've helped, David. Sometimes I'm just too sensitive."

"And I guess I'm the stereotyped temperamental neurosurgeon." He half-laughed. "I try not to be." He shifted his weight as though preparing to leave.

"Where are you from, David?"

He turned back. "Ohio. Springfield."

"Family? Brothers, sisters?"

"No," he said.

"None?"

He shook his head. "You'll be relieved to know there are no more like me. As far as I know."

She didn't understand.

"I'm an orphan," he said frankly. "Three different homes I kept running away from. I don't remember why."

"I'm sorry," she said.

"Don't be. You don't miss what you never knew."

Jennifer hesitated, but asked, "Were you ever afraid, David?"

"Sure. Who isn't?"

"Are you now?"

"No. Why?"

She chipped absently at a thumbnail. "Operating on people's brains is a big responsibility."

"So is living, if you try to do it right."

"But just living, you're only responsible for yourself. If a surgeon makes a wrong decision, somebody else suffers."

West turned her face to him, stared into her eyes for a long moment. "Is that why you're doing all these fellowships?"

She stiffened. "I want to be the best in my field."

He smiled. "It's normal to be a little frightened, Jennie. Private practice is a big responsibility."

"You're not frightened."

"I'm concerned," he said. "I work very hard to learn everything I can. If I make mistakes, they'll be beyond my control. That's all you can ask of anybody."

Jennifer leaned back and stared at the ceiling. "I envy your confidence, David. You're either very good at assuming responsibility, or you've never been really tested."

"You make it sound as though you were going into the jungles to practice. There's always somebody around to consult. Talk things out with."

She tried to force a smile. "Sure," she said. But she wanted to say: There are some things you can't ask about. You just quietly do them. Or you don't.

After West left, Jennifer leaned back against the door and closed her eyes, smelling and tasting his masculine scents and flavors. One kiss had aroused the ache deep inside her. She'd wanted to press herself against him, feel his sensuous lips on her flesh. To take him to her bed, to touch, explore, feel, to tease, and to satisfy. Most of all, to hold him close against her through the night, and kiss his stubbled mouth at morning's light. It had been so long. She shook her head to clear her mind. A man she hardly knew. Impetuous, aggressive. Almost brusque at times. Maybe because he'd grown up alone. Without a mother's influence. One minute he made her furious. And the next, he could be soft and tender, considerate, understanding.

At length Jennifer washed her hair, took a long hot bath, and fixed a cup of tea. She sat at her desk, her damp hair wrapped in a towel, and wrote a letter.

My dearest Steve,
   Though nobody will ever take your special place in my heart, I have met the most stimulating, yet most exasperating man I've ever known next to you. He's intelligent, strong, handsome, dynamic, and I really know almost nothing about him. Regardless, I wanted to make love to him tonight so badly I ache through to my bones. I think you'd like him, if you were here. But then, if you were here, I never would have met him. I am thoroughly confused. I'm sorry I let you down when you needed me so badly. I need you now.

                                   Love always,
                                        Jennifer

She carefully folded the blue sheet of stationery and dropped it in the wastebasket. Then she began the next letter.

Dear Aunt Tilda,
   Enclosed is my check for one hundred dollars. I hope you'll use it to buy something special for yourself. Something frivolous that you don't really need but have always wanted. . . .

As Jennifer hugged her pillow close against her at the edge of sleep near midnight, Lisa Waters stared wide-eyed but unseeing toward the black ceiling of her dark room, remembering the exciting sensations in her fingertips and arms. She wondered how it would feel to press a lighted cigarette against the backs of her hands, or maybe to her nipples, or her eyes. She wished she had a cigarette. She wished she smoked. If only she could get her hands free.

In the room adjacent to Lisa's, Laniet Teague managed to wedge her big toe between the metal bed frame and the side rail, despite the tight leather ankle restraints. Drenched with perspiration, she slowly maneuvered her leg to the side until she felt the toe turn and lock in place against the frame. With a sudden violent leg rotation to the left, she heard a sickening snap and felt the bone shatter and go loose. She moaned softly, the sensation almost orgasmic, and rolled her head from side to side, panting, savoring the beautiful pain while it lasted.

6

———◆◆◆———

"It's my *neck*," the strapping young man said, rubbing coarse fingers along the back of his thick neck. "Every fight, it hurts worse." He spoke in a slow, easy drawl.

Jennifer wrote down his complaints, curious about why anyone would choose to be a boxer in the first place. "What did the neurologist tell you?" she asked.

"Said it was a pinched nerve or something. In my neck bones."

She asked about similar pains in the past. There were none. Then she examined him and found him to be overly muscular, but well conditioned. In excellent health. She told him.

Kid Foster smiled a wide smile, exaggerating the curve in his crooked nose. "They say I'm the twenty-two-year-old great white hope. I'm gonna take the title."

Jennifer nodded, then explained the pain-threshold test procedure. Kid Foster readily agreed. "Nothin' much hurts me," he said, " 'cept my neck sometimes."

During Kid Foster's tests, Jennifer was amazed to see him smile and shake his head as she gradually raised him to a pain-stimulus level 12. "That doesn't hurt?"

"Kind of stings a little."

At level 16, Kid Foster nodded. "Gettin' close."

At 17 he agreed that was about how the neck pain felt.

But it had been worse after his last fight, for a couple of days. "And I had trouble liftin' my right arm. That went away."

Jennifer explained her findings to Nurse Kane, who gave Kid Foster an injection. As he started to leave, Jennifer asked, "Why do you like to fight?"

Foster grinned, lifted his broad shoulders. "I'm good at it," he drawled. "It's all I know." He left, promising to return twice a week.

Jennifer's next patient in the clinic was the old woman with shingles, number 1024, who grumbled that she had no relief from her pain whatsoever. On her tests, however, Jennifer found her pain level to be down to 6, a great improvement. And Jennifer noted that Mary, Mrs. 1024, had raised her pain threshold to more than double since her first recorded tests. The stoic old woman sucked in her prune mouth and nodded silently as Jennifer recorded her test findings. Kane took Mary into an adjacent room for her medication, and Mary left, canary legs carefully aiming her out-turned, run-over black orthopedic shoes down the hall. Jennifer was almost certain the old woman had been receiving nothing but a placebo for her pain: injections of sterile water. So West was right. It was possible to raise your pain threshold with repeated pain stimuli. The body's own endorphin system simply made more natural morphine. Jennifer was anxious to ask Dr. Neilson about other patients who might have proven the theory.

Jennifer saw her last patient before lunch, went to the reception desk to ask Nurse Kane to medicate him, but saw Kane's back turn the corner going toward the rear entrance to the lab. On an impulse, Jennifer stooped to glance under the desk, and saw the unlocked drawer with Kane's precious appointment books inside. She quickly pulled the recent book out and opened it to December appointments. She searched hurriedly for either Laniet Teague's name or code number 997. She recognized number 1024, Mary Rubens; Lisa Waters, number 1029; and Kid Foster, among others. But there was no 997. Disappointed but apprehensive, she replaced the appointment book. As she stood, Nurse Kane approached stiffly, glaring at her.

"May I ask what you're doing?"

Jennifer thought fast. "Looking for Kid Foster's chart. I forgot to note something in his history."

Kane narrowed her eyes, then glanced at the open cabinet and drawer beneath the desk. "If you can't remember to complete the charts, perhaps you should work elsewhere."

Jennifer felt her cheeks burn. "I do my job."

"And lab time is for experiments. Not socializing."

Jennifer didn't understand.

"You and Dr. West. You'd best try to concentrate on your work."

Jennifer could hold back no longer. "Look, Nurse Kane," emphasizing the *Nurse*, "what I do in my own time is my business." She started to go further, but held her tongue. "Are there any more appointments?"

Kane's expression remained cool, aloof. "Be in the lab by one o'clock."

Jennifer wheeled and marched to the elevators, glaring at a harried intern she almost bumped into as she rounded the corner.

In the cafeteria, Jennifer purposely waited for a single table in hopes David West might join her for lunch. The gigantic room was overflowing with lunching hospital personnel. She scanned the room as she began to eat. She had hoped West might drop by the clinic after surgery, but he hadn't. She spotted the pretty brunette nurse she had seen with David, her shapely legs still beneath a much-too-short uniform dress, but she ate alone. A squat gray-haired nurse with cigarette dangling from a corner of her mouth asked if she could join Jennifer.

"I'm sorry, the seat's taken," Jennifer said.

The nurse squinted one eye against her smoke and shuffled to a nearby table. Jennifer's heart leaped when she saw West appear at the side entrance to the cafeteria. She raised her hand, but he didn't see it. Just as she set her teacup on the table and stood, West flashed his white grin and walked quickly to where the pretty brunette nurse sat. Jennifer tried not to watch as the girl's face lit up when West briefly took her hand in his. Jennifer sat quickly and tried to concentrate on her salad and hard-boiled egg. When she looked again, West threw his head back and laughed at something very funny while his companion swung one pretty leg back and forth like a pendulum under the table, sharing their private joke. Minutes later, Jennifer's beeper sounded just as she set her untouched tray of food on the dirty-dish conveyor belt.

After answering her page, Jennifer went straight to the medical-staff office, curious about what they might want. A secretary asked her to take a seat until Mrs. Rogers was free. She had to wait fifteen minutes before she was called inside.

"There's been a complaint filed against you," the house-staff coordinator said.

Jennifer was flabbergasted. "For what?"

The prim, powdered, matronly woman removed her wire glasses. "Failing to complete medical records on your patients. Not taking your research projects seriously. Allowing an animal to injure itself during an experiment."

Jennifer slumped back in her chair, shaking her head. "I don't believe this. It simply isn't true."

Mrs. Rogers' face was impassive. "Then what is true?"

Jennifer didn't know where to start. It had to be Nurse Kane. She didn't want to sound paranoid, but Kane had obviously disliked her from the first day. "Mrs. Rogers, I'm afraid there's a personality conflict between myself and Nurse Kane. Nothing more. I am not negligent in my duties."

Rogers replaced her glasses, made a note on the paper on her desk, looked up again. "I must warn you, doctor. There are many applicants for research jobs. Personality conflict or no, we cannot tolerate friction in our clinics. Complaints such as this can cost you your job. I suggest you make amends." Rogers stood.

Jennifer took a deep breath, exhaled slowly. She

nodded, turned, and left. Bitch, she thought. No-good, sneaky, conniving bitch.

Finding that the rain had stopped, Jennifer took a fast outside walk along First Avenue to cool down her anger and frustration. It was still bitter cold, and she rubbed at her arms and blew into her hands when she reentered the hospital a block away. She went to the O.B. floor to look in on Maria Ortez. To her surprise, Maria was halfway down the corridor from her room, near the nursery.

"Well, you're up and around early," Jennifer said.

Maria's caramel face split into a wide smile. "I feelin' good. You see my son?"

Jennifer nodded, walking beside Maria. "He's a beautiful boy. He looks like you."

Maria giggled, cupping her hand over her mouth. "No, he more pretty than me. Very han'some. And eat? Oh, my."

"You walk like you haven't had anything done. Don't your stitches hurt?"

Maria shook her head innocently. "No hurt. Feel very good. You go see Juan now? I take you."

"I'll come back," Jennifer said. "I'm due in clinic." She clasped Maria's hand for a moment and left. She couldn't believe Maria was even out of bed. Her first child. And after an episiotomy? Jennifer cringed at the thought of cutting and enlarging the vaginal opening in performing an episiotomy, even if it did make for an easier delivery. She thought of Maria screaming hysterically in the labor room from her contractions, and of other patients she had heard complain about their stitches afterward. She became more convinced than ever that Dr. Neilson had developed something great, Opain.

As Jennifer waited for the elevator several floors above, Lisa Waters tentatively touched the pain-control button in her right hand, pressing her elbows down against the firm wooden arms of the large chair to brace herself. She felt like she was in the movies she had seen of people in old electric chairs in prison, all strapped in. Except she got to push her own button. A tingly-crawling sensation spread from her fingers along both arms, sort of tickling and teasing. She watched the red numbers on the digital screen advance slowly to 10. Something gurgled low in her abdomen. She heard her breath coming in short gasps as the number 11 lit up, and the pain moved into her shoulders and neck. Something trickled down her forehead into her right eye, blurring her vision, but it didn't sting like perspiration usually did. She closed the eye and pressed the button harder, wishing she had a cigarette. When she blinked again, the number 12 appeared before her, slightly out of focus, but it didn't matter. What mattered was that all-consuming feeling creeping up her spine, as though her back muscles had knotted into a tight ball of raw nerves, each spasm sending new bursts of pain throughout her body in concentric ripples from one central source. Her thumb blanched white as she struggled to raise the numbers higher and higher, the sound of her own teeth grating together audible above her labored breathing. "More," she heard a guttural voice demand between her gritted teeth. "More."

In the lab, Jennifer performed the experiments set up, and made notes in the appropriate books. She was only a little disappointed that David West wasn't in the lab, and greatly relieved that Nurse Kane was nowhere around. She'd have a hard time not telling Kane off, no matter how badly she needed the job. Her blood boiled from the thought of the haughty nurse, her plastic, impassive face staring down her nose at everything and everybody, never raising her dark eyebrows or mussing a peroxided hair on her superior head. Yuk.

Though uncomfortable in his presence, Jennifer tried to ignore Josef when he entered, nodding at his greeting and concentrating on her experiments. She turned once when a frantic squealing sound startled her, and saw Josef calmly lift a panic-stricken white rat from its cage. Jennifer almost cried out when the rat viciously bit Josef's wrist and clawed at his arm before he got a firm grip on the nape of its neck. Josef calmly wiped out the cage and righted a spilled water bowl, then replaced the rat. Jennifer couldn't believe he hadn't worn gloves. And he hadn't even seemed to notice the bites and scratches. When he glanced down at the blood trickling across his wrist, he licked it off and went to the next cage.

"You should irrigate that wound," Jennifer said. "And sterilize it." She walked to his side.

"It's okay, doctor."

She took his hand and inspected the torn flesh. The teeth marks were deep puncture wounds, already clotting. "When was your last tetanus shot?"

He stared off into space for a moment. "Nurse Kane give me one two years ago, I think."

"You'll need another. Come over here." She flushed out the wound with peroxide and with sterile saline. Josef agreed to go to the emergency room for the tetanus shot, and she called to arrange it. At three-fifteen, Jennifer took a call from the gynecology clinic, agreed to see a patient right away.

Ella Lu Mavis arrived in the Pain Control Clinic in a wheelchair. A stick-thin black girl with a big head and wide brown eyes, doubled over in pain, her cheeks wet and salt-streaked from her own tears. Diagnosis, PID, acute pelvic inflammatory disease, secondary to gonorrhea. Between sobs, Ella Lu said she was eighteen, and this was the third time she'd had "the PID'S."

Jennifer went over the girl's gynecology records quickly. She was on Ampicillin to control the infection, but neither codeine nor Percodan had eased her pain. Jennifer examined her, but Ella Lu would hardly allow her to touch the skin over her lower abdomen, near her ovaries. The right side was especially tender, she said.

"Have you had your appendix out?" Jennifer asked.

"No. Ain't nobody gonna cut on me."

Jennifer nodded. "Ella Lu, you've got to get this cleared up. And stop catching it. If you had an acute appendicitis, nobody would ever know."

Ella Lu looked away, her expression bored.

"It can make you sterile, too. Don't you want children someday?"

Ella Lu winced and withdrew as Jennifer pressed gently over her right side. "Ain't interested in no babies," she mumbled, her face drawn.

At length Jennifer wrote out her findings and took the chart to Nurse Kane's desk. Kane virtually ignored her, and, without a word, drew up an injection for Ella Lu. Jennifer watched through the open door to the medication room, noted that the injection came from a box numbered three. Other numbered boxes sat side by side on the same shelf. Before Kane could turn around, Jennifer returned to the lab.

As Jennifer prepared to repeat the pain-threshold experiments on the two white sister rats, she noticed a black spot on the top of one rat's head. She looked closer to be sure. Josef returned from the emergency room, his hand neatly bandaged in white gauze.

"Josef, did you change these rats since yesterday?"

"No, ma'am."

She looked again. "But this one has a black spot. It wasn't there before."

He ambled over and looked. "Must be dirt."

"No, it's black hair." She tried to read his large, vacant eyes.

He shook his head. "Musta been there, then. It's the same rat." He went to the back of the lab.

Jennifer followed him. "What did you do with the rat that went bonkers?"

"Bonkers?"

"The one that kept crashing his head against the cage."

Josef scooped rat food out of a bag into a cup. "Oh, him. He's all right."

"Where is he?"

Josef began to distribute the food to the animals. "In back. With the monkeys."

"Monkeys?"

He nodded. "He's okay. Just went cage-crazy."

"You've seen it before?"

He straightened from where he bent over a cage, stared down at her. "Why do you want to know?"

"Just curious. I don't know much about animals."

"It happens sometimes. He'll be okay." He turned and left the room through a rear door, locking it behind him.

Jennifer began the experiment on the two rats, repeating exactly what David West had done, following his notations in the lab notebook. But something was wrong. The rat with the black spot squealed and raced about frantically at a pain setting of 3, while it had ignored the pain almost to a level of 7 in West's experiment. She double-checked her results. No question about it. Somebody had exchanged this rat for the other. But who? Why?

When Jennifer finished in the lab, she retrieved her purse and sweater, went to see Melanie Wardner.

"How are you feeling?" she asked.

Melanie stretched her arms over her head as if yawning, quickly scooted up in the raised-back bed. "Great. How 'bout you?"

Jennifer said she was fine. A quick look at Melanie's chart told her Melanie had received absolutely no pain or sleep medication for the past twenty-four hours. Jennifer noticed a Kleenex bandage on one of Melanie's fingers. "What happened there?"

"Oh, that. I guess I pinched it in the side rails." She quickly covered it with her other hand. "It's nothing."

"Let me see," Jennifer said, reaching for her hand.

Melanie pulled back. "Really. It's nothing."

Jennifer insisted. When she looked, she almost got sick. The entire pad of flesh at the tip of Melanie's index finger was crushed and black, peeled back from the dead-white bone. A quivering black blood clot fell from the crushed skin, splatted on Jennifer's white shoe.

"This is terrible," Jennifer declared. "You could lose this finger."

Melanie cocked her head to one side and grinned. "It doesn't hurt."

Jennifer quickly called Dr. Bevins, who arranged for a plastic-surgery consult. Later, Jennifer watched as the plastic surgeon created a flap of skin to cover the raw, exposed fingertip. But she couldn't understand why Melanie insisted on having the surgery performed without any anesthesia. The surgeon said there must be nerve damage to render the area so numb. When he explored the nerves of the finger, they were intact and normal. Melanie left the operating room in good spirits, smiling, and happier than Jennifer had seen her before. The surgeon said he had never known anybody so brave in twenty years of practice.

Jennifer peeked in the nursery through the observation window on her way downstairs, and spoke briefly with the nurse on duty.

"Best baby we've had in ages," the nurse said.

"He is cute," Jennifer agreed. "His mother's very proud of him."

"Proud? That's not the word. She's here ten, twelve times a day to see him. He never cries, that one. Wet, dirty, hungry, doesn't matter. I wish they were all that good."

Jennifer agreed, made a brief note in Juan's chart, and headed for home. As she started out the front door, she stopped short. On the First Avenue sidewalk, the leggy brunette nurse wove her arm around David West's, gazing up into his smiling face as they walked toward Jennifer. At that instant, someone touched her shoulder.

"Can I buy you that drink now?" Dr. Neilson asked.

She glanced quickly toward David West, then into Neilson's distinguished face. "I'd love it." She put her arm in Neilson's, and barely nodded as they passed West and his nurse seconds later.

"Tell me about yourself," Neilson said when they were seated at Maxwell's Plum Restaurant.

Jennifer glanced out the frosted window from their sidewalk seat at rushing passersby puffing their little clouds of steam in the cold air. "There isn't much to tell." She looked back into his deep blue eyes, alert, intelligent, and bemused.

Neilson removed his glasses and put them in his coat pocket. "You're about twenty-seven, maybe twenty-eight years old. Slight Southern accent. A very pretty

young woman. Bright. About five-feet-five, I'd say.
Maybe a hundred ten, twelve pounds. Good figure,
though you try to hide it. Full, sensuous lips. A little
hitch in your walk, proud. Brown eyes with tiny gold
flecks at the edges. Sincere, trusting eyes. And warm,
like a doe. Shall I go on?"

She almost blushed. "I'd rather you didn't. What
about you?"

The waiter interrupted their conversation briefly, took
the order. Neilson smiled, tiny laugh lines around his
eyes adding a few years to his face, more in keeping
with his silver temples. "I'm a thoroughly obsessed neu-
rophysiologist M.D.," he said. "Determined to free the
world of pain."

"A noble cause."

He wafted the compliment away with one hand. "I'm
overworked, underpaid, often lonely, and I miss the
company of beautiful women. Aside from that, I'm a totally dedicated, perfectionistic bastard."

When their wine arrived, Jennifer clinked her glass to
his. "To pain," she said. "Without it, you would have no
cause." They drank.

"As quixotic as you make me sound, my windmills are
real."

"And universal," Jennifer said. "Nondiscriminatory.
Who among you has never experienced pain?"

Neilson toyed with his wineglass absently. "It is not a
subject I take lightly."

"I'm not making fun. I've read your papers. Seen your
results. You're very good."

Neilson exhaled a short sigh, leaned forward with arms
folded on the table. "And I asked about you. Background, family, interests, romantic status."

Jennifer sipped her Chablis. It *was* better than what
she normally bought. "No family, except an aunt. From
Atlanta. My first love is reconstructive surgery. The others are my two goldfish and African violets, but they
won't bloom in the cold weather."

"You left one out."

She squared her napkin beside the ashtray. "Romantic status, zero."

A faint smile tugged at the corners of his mouth. "We have something in common." They laughed.

"I'm truly amazed at the results with Opain," Jennifer said.

Neilson's face became serious. "It's sometimes hard to believe just how good it is."

She thought of the rat battering itself against the cage. "Any problems with it?" She tried to sound nonchalant.

"Nothing serious." His pupils changed almost imperceptibly.

"Do you remember a girl named Laniet Teague? Young, pretty, with red hair?"

His expression didn't change. "Doesn't ring a bell. I'm sure I'd remember from your description. Though I prefer hair long and brown. Something like yours."

Jennifer's beeper sounded, causing people at nearby tables to interrupt their conversations, turn toward the strange noise.

"Excuse me," she said, and went to the phone downstairs.

When she returned, she apologized for the interruption, said a patient had asked for her in the emergency room.

Neilson stood, offered to walk her back. She declined.

"Another time, then. For dinner?"

"Sounds good. Anytime." They shook hands.

On her hurried walk back to New Hope University Hospital, Jennifer reevaluated Dr. Neilson. There was a warm, personal side to the man, unlike many researchers. She'd seen it at Melanie Wardner's bedside when Melanie was screaming in agony in the recovery room. And again with Maria Ortez in the labor room. He projected compassion. Yet there was something very lonely about the man. Almost vulnerable. He was quite handsome, distinguished, and accomplished. Yes, she decided. She would enjoy having dinner with Neilson. Very much. And David West could just keep his pretty little nurse.

When she entered the medicinal-smelling emergency

room, the charge nurse told her quickly about the patient. "Room three. Name's Jackson. Walter. Throat cancer. He's oozing blood down his neck."

"Oh, my God," Jennifer shouted. "Get me a head-and-neck tray fast. And emergency consult. His carotid artery's about to blow."

7

Jennifer raced past frenetic nurses and doctors to emergency room three. Walter Jackson sat on the vinyl exam table holding a blood-soaked handkerchief to his bloated neck, thin wisps of white hair not quite hiding his scalp. His sallow skin was drawn so tightly over his facial bones, he resembled a skull painted with pale acrylic flesh tones. His eyes were as sunken as Jennifer remembered, watery blue, but seemed to focus on her this time. A smile spread his lips, exposing half-rotted, tobacco-stained teeth uncared for over many years. "I wanted to thank you," he began weakly.

"Don't talk." Jennifer lifted the handkerchief from his neck. The nauseating smell of long-dead meat filled her nostrils where the grayish-white grainy cancer crater ate through his skin. Lumpy yellow pus and saliva dribbled from the core of the open sore, mixing with a trickling stream of crimson blood. Jennifer ripped open the head-and-neck pack, barked orders to a nurse for an intravenous line and emergency type and cross-match of six units of blood.

Jackson caught her wrist, shook his shrunken head slowly from side to side as much as the massive malignancy in his neck would allow. "No," he said. "It's over."

75

Jennifer could smell the raw whiskey on his breath.

He chuckled hoarsely. "I'm not afraid to go anymore. You took away the pain." He coughed, suddenly increasing the erratic stream of blood from his ulcerating neck to a small river of red, draining his life away. "Can I smoke?" he asked.

"Not in here," the nurse said.

Jennifer reached into the old man's open shirt pocket and took out his last two cigarettes. She put one in his mouth, one in hers. Lifting the book of matches from his shaking fingers, she lit them both. She nodded at the stunned nurse, closed the door when the nurse exited. Jennifer sat on the stool opposite Walter Jackson and tried to smoke, watching the river of blood clot beneath his frayed shirt collar and drip onto his stained khaki pants.

"Drink?" he asked.

"Sure." She opened the offered half-pint and took a small swig, passing it back to him.

He took a long draw at the bottle, recapped it.

"Mmm, that's good," he said, hugging the bottle to his chest like a lover's keepsake. His color faded faster than a broken thermometer.

"Would you like to lie down?" Jennifer asked.

He nodded, still smiling. "Maybe I better."

Jennifer helped him swing his scrawny legs up on the table. His ankles were ringed black where socks should have been, his battered shoes untied. She balled a fresh towel and held it to his neck.

"I just didn't want to go alone," he whispered, touching her hand.

"I'm here." Jennifer's eyes stung and her vision blurred till she could hardly see his smiling face. She took the cigarette from his lips, flicked the ash on the floor, and replaced it. Just then, his carotid artery blew out with the force of Vesuvius, an inch-diameter hose, shooting a pulsating stream of blood to the acoustical ceiling and spattering the white wall red near where he lay. Jennifer closed her eyes when his warm blood struck her full in the face, but took his hand in hers and squeezed. "I'm here, Walter," she whispered.

Jackson opened his eyes only once more. "It don't hurt."

Sometime later, when the door opened, Jennifer raised her head from her arm where she sat beside Walter Jackson's body.

"Jesus," the resident exclaimed.

She nodded, wiping her eyes with a corner of her sleeve.

"Carotid blowout. I've never seen one really blow."

Jennifer stood, glanced at her blood-soaked white uniform in the wall mirror, saw a gelatinous clot hanging from her spattered face, another in her hair. "You're lucky," she said, turned, and went home.

On Thursday, Jennifer managed to drag through her morning patients despite her lack of sleep. She had sat in the dark at her steamy third-floor window till dawn, staring out at the immense city, wondering how many Walter Jacksons there were in the world. And how many had to die alone. She wondered if, perhaps, that was the greatest pain of all.

One man, a successful business executive with a computer company, arrived on a stretcher, unable to move because of severe pain in his back. He told her he had ruptured a disk when he fell on an icy sidewalk in front of his apartment building six months earlier. He had tried everything for relief, including acupuncture.

"I've got to work," he said. "With inflation the way it is, everything more expensive every day. I've got three kids in college."

Jennifer said she understood. Mr. Dunlevy tested out at pain level 14. By going for a chart at just the right moment, Jennifer watched Nurse Kane select his injection from box number three: Opain. Jennifer assured Mr. Dunlevy he'd feel better very soon.

At noon, Jennifer realized neither Lisa Waters nor Ella

Lu Mavis had kept their appointments. Despite her reluctance to have another discussion with Nurse Kane, she asked if they had called to cancel.

"Mavis is obviously unreliable," Kane said. "I don't show an appointment for the other one."

Jennifer leaned forward toward the open appointment book. "I'm sure she had one. I told her Thursday."

Kane calmly closed the book. "Oh, the blond girl."

"Right. Short, little turned-up nose."

"She had to go out of town, as I recall. Won't be back for several weeks."

"Strange," Jennifer said mostly to herself. "She was looking for a job."

"Maybe she found one. Out of town."

Jennifer turned to leave, stopped. "Do you have their phone numbers?"

Kane stiffened. "No, I don't."

"They'd be in the chart. On the form they fill out."

Kane's icy stare fixed Jennifer. "I'll check."

Several minutes later, Nurse Kane brought Ella Lu Mavis' phone number into the exam room where Jennifer finished her paperwork. "The Waters girl took her records with her. I remember now."

Jennifer took the piece of paper. "Wasn't she in the study?"

"No."

"Sure she was. Number one-oh-two-something."

Kane flushed momentarily. "You're quite mistaken. She was never in the study." She wheeled and left.

Jennifer went to check on Melanie Wardner before lunch. She didn't understand why the bed was empty, and asked the floor nurse.

"She's in surgery. Stupid girl."

"But why? She was fine yesterday."

"Pulled out her catheter during the night. Without deflating the balloon. She tore her bladder stitches out."

Jennifer's heart sank. Just the thought of the pain from doing such a thing made her weak. She said she'd look in later, added, "Poor girl comes in for a little urethral dilitation, winds up with a ruptured bladder, a ripped-off fingertip, now another ruptured bladder. Two major abdominal surgeries." She couldn't believe such luck.

After lunch, Jennifer went to the lab, where she was surprised to see that David West had already begun the afternoon experiments. She coolly returned his exuberant greeting, wondering if he would ask about her evening with Neilson. He didn't.

"That's not very friendly," he said.

"I'm not in a very friendly mood. What do we do with these monsters?"

"The chimps? Same as always, but different. They're smarter." He seemed too preoccupied to notice her gray disposition.

She watched as he set up the experiment. The chimpanzees were wired like always, ears, encephalograph wires, blood pressure, pulse and respiration monitors.

"Watch," West said, pressing the control button on cage one, pain level 3. The chimp jumped up in the air, chattered noisily, waddled to a plastic lever in its cage, and pressed it down. As liquid squirted into its water bowl, the other chimp immediately shrieked, spun around twice, and raced to press the lever in its cage. When it did, liquid squirted into its water bowl and that of chimp number one, who quickly drank it and sat looking at its mate, near-human hands encircling the bars of the cage. Seconds later, the first chimp jumped and shrieked noisily, ran over and pulled the lever down again, causing the same pain reaction and events from chimp number two.

"They're wired opposite," West said. "Chimp one zaps chimp two with pain by pulling his lever. Chimp two reacts by pulling his lever, zapping chimp one, gets a reward, something for his pain. Chimp one is rewarded by zapping number two. They're almost like people. Sometimes I think they just get pissed and zap each other to get even."

Jennifer sat beside West. "What's the point?"

"One gets drug A in the bowl. The other gets drug B.

Or water. It's a direct comparison of drug effectiveness. Each zap goes up one point on the pain scale. The idea is for one to go to its tolerance level before the other. One may reach it at ten or twelve, the other at fifteen or twenty. The difference is caused by the difference in the drugs. Got it?"

Jennifer shook her head. "I think so, but I don't like it. If one had a better drug, he might kill the other one. Take him past his viable tolerance."

West grinned. "That's why we're here." He raised his eyebrows. "Can you imagie what one human might do to another if they both had zap buttons?"

She couldn't resist the opening. "They do it all the time, David."

He let out a long sigh, shoulders slumped. "Yeah."

West stopped the test before either chimpanzee became overly excited, asked Josef to return them to their cages in the rear. "I've been thinking about what you asked the other night, about patients disappearing."

Jennifer's ears perked up.

"The only one I remember was a guy with a brain tumor. I had him scheduled for surgery."

"And?"

"And he went poof. Dropped out of sight. Never came back."

"Did you try to call him?"

"Sure. Lots of times. He never answered."

"Do you remember his name? Phone number?"

"Hey, what gives?"

"Do you?"

"Sure. At home, in my case book."

Jennifer wasn't sure what gave. But she was very curious. "Did he ever come to the pain clinic?"

West thought for a moment. "Once. About a week before we'd planned his surgery. Why?"

She stood. "Never mind why. When can I get his name and number?"

"I'll bring it by tonight. Your apartment. Okay?" West's animated face broke into a grin.

"Fine," Jennifer said evenly. "If I'm not there, leave it on my desk. I believe you know how to get in."

Josef only nodded as Jennifer walked past him toward the door. She stopped for a quick look at his hand. "Looks good, Josef, but keep it clean. And dry."

"Yes, ma'am."

On the hospital's fourteenth floor, Jennifer learned that Melanie Wardner was still in the recovery room. When she arrived there, she found Melanie sleepy but apparently comfortable. The nurse said she was stable.

Jennifer leaned over the bed, brushed damp strands of hair off the girl's brow. "I'm so sorry, Melanie."

Melanie opened uncertain eyes, tried to find Jennifer's face. "Feel so good," she whispered.

"You'll feel better in the morning," Jennifer said, aware that the anesthetic limited the girl's speech.

Melanie barely nodded. " 'Swonderful." And she fell asleep.

In her apartment, Jennifer got Ella Lu Mavis' number on the second try.

"This be her mother, Mrs. Mavis," a gospel-singing voice announced. "What you want with her?"

Jennifer told her. "Is she there?"

Jennifer heard muffled voices in the background; then the phone clunked against something. "She say she don't want no operation. Won't come to the phone."

"Can you tell me where you live?"

"Honey, I'll tell you, but it won't do no good. Ella Lu done made up her mind. She don't listen to me, she sure not gonna listen to you."

Jennifer finally got the address. "It's not about surgery," she said. "I just want to talk to her."

At eight-fifteen that evening, Jennifer got off the bus on West Ninety-fourth Street and walked the two blocks to the address Mrs. Mavis had given her. Dark faces stared sullenly at her from doorways, but the biting cold of the blustery night had cleared the streets of all but an occasional straggler. They, too, seemed in a hurry. Jennifer rang the bell to apartment three-C in the tiny vestibule beside graffiti-covered mailboxes, but nothing happened. Finally she climbed the three flights of narrow stairs, careful not to rub against the soot-blackened wall, long devoid of even flaking paint. The landing on level two was dark, but light from a naked bulb on the third floor made it barely possible to pick her way. The stairs smelled of urine. The first two third-floor doors she saw had no numbers visible, just spray-painted names and crude insults.

Though the metal C was twisted, Jennifer found what she hoped was Ella Lu's apartment. She knocked, softly at first, then loud enough to be heard above the television set's canned laughter beyond the door.

The door opened about two inches as the white of a large round eye confirmed her identity from the darkness inside. Then she was admitted. Ella Lu sat yoga-style on a precariously leaning sofa in front of the television, all skinny arms, legs, and elbows. Jennifer joined her while Mrs. Mavis, a round-cheeked overweight woman with enormous haunches, busied herself in the small kitchen nearby.

"Ain't having no operation," Ella Lu said to the TV.

Jennifer explained why she had come. "How's your pain?"

Ella Lu shrugged her narrow shoulders. "Okay."

"What's okay? A little better? A lot?"

The thin black girl stared straight ahead, her head balanced on her scrawny neck like an olive on a toothpick. "Gone."

"The pain's completely gone?" Jennifer asked.

Ella Lu turned to look at her as if she were deaf. "I said gone."

"Can you come by the pain clinic sometime this week?"

"I already said no."

Jennifer moved forward to try to see her eyes. "I haven't asked before."

"That nurse did."

Jennifer felt herself tighten, her senses alert. "Which nurse?"

"The one don't like me. Ol' stoneface."

Jennifer sat farther forward. "Nurse Kane?"

"I guess. She jabbed me with that needle. She didn' have to do it so hard." She turned to face Jennifer, her large eyes accusing.

Jennifer tried to lock her stare. "When did you tell her you wouldn't come back?"

Ella Lu turned back to the old movie. "When she call."

Jennifer fought to retain her patience. "When did she call?"

" 'Bout twelve-fifteen. During the news."

Confused and irritated, Jennifer said she'd be glad to see Ella Lu if her pain came back, excused herself, and left. On the windy street outside, she suddenly felt foolish for making the trip. A victim of her own imagination. Ella Lu was perfectly all right. Jennifer felt uncomfortable on the dark street alone, and quickened her pace, her heels echoing against the dim buildings. With no taxis in sight, she walked back toward the bus stop, pulling her coat tightly around her, the collar up around her neck.

At West Ninety-fifth Street she became aware of soft footfalls behind her, gradually closing the distance between them. She didn't dare turn to look, but shifted her weight to the balls of her feet and forced her steps still faster. The footfalls quickened almost at the same time. Without moving her head, she searched both sides of the empty street for a lighted store, a bar, church, some place to enter. Everything was locked up for the night. She crossed to the opposite side of the street, almost in a trot, and purposely walked beneath the misty streetlight, planning to look back when the footsteps would be under the light and she in the shadows. She strained to hear the soft scuffing sounds of feet above the pulse thundering in her ears. When she was twenty feet beyond the light, she turned quickly. Nobody was there. Something moved in a shadowed doorway across the street, then stood perfectly still, merging with the dark. Was it the outline of a man? Or her imagination? She turned quickly to hurry on her way and almost screamed when something jumped out of the shadows ahead and a horrid clattering noise pierced the night. Her heart pounded almost through her ribs as she watched a huge rat dart out from under a toppled garbage-can lid and across the street into an alley. She broke into an all-out run for Eighth Avenue, unable to hear whether anybody ran behind her. At the corner, she saw a taxi unloading a passenger, and dived into the open rear door almost before the passenger was out.

In front of her apartment, she paid the driver with cold hands trembling so badly she could hardly remove the change from her purse, and ran inside. She didn't notice the taxi that pulled up across the street as she entered her building, or its occupant, who watched her hasty retreat.

Upstairs, Jennifer unlocked her door, flipped on the lights before entering, then slammed and locked the door and leaned against it to catch her breath and let her heart slow. She felt chilled to the bone. She put water on to boil, undressed and put on her robe, and ran into the bathroom for a hot shower. By the time she had dried herself after the shower, the teakettle had almost boiled dry. Refilling it, she thought she heard something at her door, like a soft scuffing of shoes. She froze, breathless, waiting, listening. It scuffed again. She tiptoed to the door, teakettle in hand, and turned off the light. A shadow moved from outside, visible along the crack at the bottom of the door. Suddenly something brushed against her bare foot, and she jumped back, screamed, and dropped the kettle.

Her doorknob turned before she could speak, and the door burst open. "What's wrong?" David West demanded.

Too weak to speak, Jennifer threw her arms around his solid arms and back and buried her face against his chest. When she had calmed herself, she explained the events of the evening as they sat on the sofa, her body tucked close against his.

"I came by earlier," West said, "but you weren't here. So I came back to bring you my patient's name, the one with the brain tumor. I decided to slip it under the door instead of breaking and entering again."

"Thank God it was you."

He kissed her forehead, spoke softly. "Well, do I stay tonight, or go back in the freezing cold?"

She sat up, studying his earnest face. "David, it wouldn't be fair to you."

"Let me decide that."

She shook her head. "I'm serious. I'd give anything to have you stay. But only to hold. To be close. I'm not ready for more."

After a while he grinned his lazy grin. "It beats sleeping alone."

When Jennifer was almost asleep, curled against his strong back, West asked, "Who's Steve?"

She felt herself tense, but pulled him tighter to her. "Not now," she said.

The night-nursery nurse checked her newborns for wet diapers, the last check before their morning feedings. She picked up little Juan Belmondo Ortez, soaking wet but uncomplaining. "This is the best baby," she said, handing him to her aide.

The nurse's aide quickly changed Juan's diaper, safety pins in her mouth from habit. She dropped a can of talcum just as she almost fastened the second pin on his dry diaper. She replaced Juan Ortez into his bassinet and carefully tucked the blue blanket around his sides. Little Juan kicked his legs a few times as the sharp point of the pin pierced his thin brown skin, and pursed his lips in the sucking reflex. When he kicked again, the pin drove itself deeper into his flesh. He wasn't old enough to smile. He sucked at his lips. But he didn't cry.

8

＊＊＊——◆——＊＊＊

When Jennifer awakened at seven A.M. Friday to answer the phone, David West was gone, the crumpled pillow beside her the only evidence he'd been there. She fumbled for the phone, managed a hello.

"Please be in the medical-staff office at eight," the secretary said.

Jennifer downed a piece of toast and cup of tea as she dressed, and raced across a freezing First Avenue toward the hospital amid hordes of rushing uniformed hospital employees.

"These are very serious charges," Mrs. Rogers said, peering over her round glasses from behind her uncluttered desk.

Jennifer glanced at Mrs. Rogers' college and graduate-school degrees framed on the wall behind her, and her registered nurse's certificate. The one charge was almost too ludicrous to discuss. The other too painful. "He was dying, Mrs. Rogers. Terminal cancer."

Rogers glanced at the paper in her hand. "You ignored the restriction on smoking in the emergency room. You knew there was oxygen nearby."

Jennifer sighed. "An old man wanted a cigarette before he died."

"And you partook of whiskey with him? It was reported on your breath."

Jennifer pushed at a cuticle with her fingernail, looked up into the prim woman's small eyes. "Yes."

Rogers' stern expression hardened like setting plaster. "Instead of making an effort to save the patient's life, you sat down, had a drink and cigarette, and watched him bleed to death."

Jennifer felt her anger rising. "He had terminal cancer. Incurable. His doctors had given up."

"And you took it on yourself to make that decision? To decide it was time for him to die?"

Jennifer shook her head, her eyes stinging at the memory. "It was his decision," she said huskily.

Rogers cleared her turkey-gobbler throat. "We do not condone euthanasia at New Hope, doctor. Nor ignoring hospital regulations. Consider yourself suspended as of this moment. You'll have a medical-staff board hearing next week."

Jennifer stood, swallowed at a lump in her throat. "Mrs. Rogers, how much time have you spent recently taking care of patients? Lonely old men, suffering children?"

Rogers bristled. "I am a registered nurse."

"With a tidy little desk, sharp pencils, and a clipboard. It's easy to make judgments from behind a desk, after the fact. I suggest you spend a month in the children's wing of the cancer unit, or on the radiotherapy ward. Then file your report to the medical-staff board." Jennifer grabbed her shoulder bag and stormed out of the office.

In the hall outside, she leaned against the wall and cried, ignoring curious but silent passersby. She found a women's rest room, finally washed her puffy face in cold water, and walked up to the Pain Control Clinic to tell them to cancel her appointments.

Nurse Kane stood rigidly behind her reception counter as Jennifer approached. Almost more than being suspended, Jennifer dreaded the indignity of having to admit it to Kane.

"What do you want?" Kane quipped. "You're suspended."

Jennifer felt her blood pressure rise inside her skull. "How do you know?"

Kane never blinked. "It's common knowledge. I should think you can forget your plastic fellowship now as well." Kane turned and called for the first patient, one of three waiting on the benches, leaving Jennifer alone.

Jennifer swung the leather bag's strap over her shoulder and started to leave.

"Jennie, wait." David West almost jogged down the hall. He took her arm and kept moving, forcing her to run to keep up with his long strides. She tried to tell him about losing her job.

"I heard. I got a great case in surgery this morning. Come on, you'll love it."

Once she changed into her green scrub dress and entered the operating room, Jennifer felt at home again. Human. She watched as three surgeons and two scrub nurses prepared the deformed twelve-year-old boy for surgery to move his eyes closer together. She studied the boy's photographs and X rays taped to a lighted viewbox on one wall. His eyes were so far apart they appeared to be on stalks, like an insect's, and his nose was correspondingly broad between. Hypertelorism. She'd seen only one such case before.

West winked one dark eye at Jennifer through the slit between his green cap and mask as she approached the operating table. The familiar rhythmic sighs of the bellows of the anesthesia machine were like music to Jennifer's ears, somehow underlining the seriousness of the job at hand. West introduced her quickly to the others.

"Ah, Jennifer," the tall surgeon in front of her said, turning.

"Dr. Bronson," she said respectfully, amazed to see the chief of Plastic Surgery scrubbed on the case.

For the next two hours she watched every move the surgeons made, quickly raising the scalp from the patient's head, opening the front of the skull, lifting the frontal lobes of the youngster's brain. David West

worked quickly and silently to that point, his dark eyes
flashing in total concentration, his hands smooth and
deft, gentle. Under Bronson's supervision, the plastic-surgery resident divided the bones around the boy's eyes.
Jennifer savored the sweet-burned smell of saw blade
against bone as they removed enough bone from the
nose to move the eye sockets close to their normal posi-
tions. Bronson wasn't totally satisfied with the correction, said so. He turned to Jennifer. "You're a nose
specialist, Barton. What do you think? Can we get them
closer together?"

She studied the correction again. "If you remove the
rest of each ethmoid sinus, you can."

Bronson nodded, turned back. "Do it," he said.

Jennifer was flattered, though she knew Bronson had
known exactly what to do. He was merely making his
point.

After surgery, Jennifer told West, "You're a damned
good neurosurgeon."

He winked at her. "I try." West had to scrub on another case, so Jennifer changed into her whites and
started for the fourteenth floor to see Melanie Wardner.
Her beeper sounded, interrupting her plans.

On the phone, Neilson said, "I don't care what Nurse
Rogers said, I need help in the clinic. Get down here."

Jennifer went to the clinic, ignored Nurse Kane's
glare, and went to work. Kid Foster came in a little after
noon. "How's the neck?" Jennifer asked.

"Like it ain't there," he drawled, illustrating by lolling
his head around a three-sixty circle.

On the pain-threshold machine, she found his cervical
pain to be totally absent, while his threshold for pain had
risen to level twenty. Opain had done it again. Foster
thanked her, asked if she'd like tickets to his next fight.

"Thanks anyway," Jennifer replied. "It's a little too
brutal for me."

He nodded. "Yeah. My girl don't go, either."

At twelve-thirty, Doctor Neilson stopped Jennifer
outside her examining room. "Jennie, can you possibly

do the experiments alone this afternoon? West is tied up, and I've got something that can't wait. It's urgent."

She reminded him of her suspension.

"This is more important. I'll speak with the medical-staff office."

After a quick lunch, Jennifer performed the experiments as requested. To her surprise, the sister rats appeared to be the original pair she had seen West work with. There was no black spot on either's head. And the test results were identical to the ones West had obtained. Something funny was going on. But what? She didn't mention it to Josef.

At two-thirty, she interrupted her experiments long enough to dial the phone number of Arnold Heath, the brain-tumor patient David West had told her about. A woman's voice answered.

"Is this some kind of sick joke?" the woman asked.

Jennifer explained she was from the hospital. A doctor.

"He's dead." The woman's voice cracked, full of emotion.

"But how? When?"

Jennifer finally learned that the woman with the quavering voice on the phone was Arnold Heath's mother, that her son had died months before on the Major Degan Expressway. The police had called it suicide.

"He wouldn't commit suicide," Mrs. Heath sobbed. "Not Arnold."

Jennifer tried to ask more questions, her heart pouring out to the broken woman on the phone.

"They said he just laid down. Let the cars run over him. But he wouldn't. He'd have been too scared."

Jennifer tried to express her sympathy to the distraught mother, apologized for upsetting her, and hung up. After three tries she reached the proper highway-patrol office, and held the silent phone while a clerk looked up the records.

"A witness says he just laid down at the edge of the road with his legs on the pavement. No telling how many cars ran over him. There was blood smeared for over four hundred yards, where he was dragged and bumped along on the pavement. Identified by a card in his wallet. Only way possible, I guess. Report says he was pulverized from head to toe."

Jennifer hung up, held her head in her hands, and stared at the lab desk, upset, confused. Minutes later, she asked the Manhattan information operator for the number of Lisa Waters.

"There are over twenty Lisa or L. Waterses listed," the operator said. "What address?"

Jennifer said she didn't know and hung up. As she turned, Josef grinned his horrible grin and set a caged rat on the table behind her. Jennifer immediately saw the crusted blood on the rat's nose as it sat calmly watching her.

"That's the one that went bonkers," she exclaimed.

Josef nodded. "Cage-crazy," he said. "Told you he was all right."

She couldn't believe it. The little animal appeared perfectly normal except for his scrapes and bruises. "What did you do? He looks fine."

Josef shook his head. "Dr. Neilson gave him something, I guess."

At four-thirty, Jennifer left the lab to check on Melanie Wardner. Her knees went rubbery when she entered Melanie's room. She held to the bedside rail, stunned at what she saw. Melanie lay spread-eagled beneath the sheets on her back as though she were staked out, arms and legs tightly secured to the four corners of the bed, her face crazed and straining. A tape-padded wooden tongue blade was tightly bound between her teeth, muffling her garbled grunts of effort.

Jennifer turned to the private-duty nurse, who rose from her chair, demanded an explanation.

"She keeps trying to pull out her catheter again," the blue-haired nurse sweetly said. "And she bites her tongue. The psychiatrist said it's a reaction to the shock she's been through. Temporary."

"Psychiatrist?"

Blue-hair nodded, placid and secure, smelling of lavender bath salts. "She wasn't adequately prepared. Psychologically, you know."

Jennifer dabbed perspiration from Melanie's flushed forehead and temples with a tissue, tried to get her to focus on her face. "Melanie?" she called softly. But Melanie saw only something in her own head or far off in space. Jennifer chewed at her own lower lip, momentarily closed her eyes in disbelief, and turned. "I'll look in tomorrow." She gave her home number to the nurse, asked her to call if there was any change.

On the O.B. ward, Maria Ortez's dark eyes flashed fire. "I gonna sue the hospital," Maria declared. "To let my son stick with the pins." She paced the four-bedded room like an enraged tiger, often uttering words in Spanish Jennifer couldn't define, but understood. The other three women were wide-eyed but silent in their beds.

Jennifer got the explanation in bits and pieces, finally went to check on Juan herself. The nurse assured her the pediatrician had checked Juan thoroughly. His wound was not serious, and he was on antibiotics to halt any infection. His newborn passive immunity from his mother would prevent any serious complications. Jennifer returned to reassure Maria.

Maria paced and listened, arms folded tight against her chest. She stopped, looked at Jennifer. "Tomorrow I takin' my Juan home. They say I can't do. You watch."

On the way out, Jennifer copied Maria's home phone number and address into her address book. In case she did leave the hospital against orders, Jennifer wanted to be able to check on the two of them.

It was after five when Jennifer hurriedly unlocked her apartment door to answer the phone ringing inside.

"You seem determined to be dismissed," Mrs. Rogers said. "Seeing patients when you've been suspended is a serious infraction of regulations."

"But Dr. Neilson needed help." Jennifer could almost see the doughy woman's prim face through the phone. Overly powdered. Dry.

"Dr. Neilson doesn't make the rules. Until further notice, you are off duty without pay. You are not to enter the hospital. Be in my office Monday morning at eight."

Jennifer fumed and paced for twenty minutes after the call. She tried to reach Neilson by phone, was told he was away for the weekend. She needed to ask him to speak with the medical-staff board. More important, she had to tell him about Melanie Wardner's deteriorating condition. David West didn't answer his phone either. Jennifer finally poured herself a glass of wine, determined to regain her control.

At eight-thirty that evening, Jennifer sat on her sofa bed in robe and slippers with the voluminous Manhattan phone book open in her lap. She dialed the first L. Waters listed. Seconds later, she apologized to Larry Waters and dialed the second number. By ten-thirty she had called twenty-seven numbers without success. One man invited her over for a drink and "a little private party" before she hung up. Another tried to sell her life insurance. Three phones had been disconnected with no new numbers. Two didn't answer. She kept trying those two.

A freezing, blowing rain clattered against Jennifer's window at eleven P.M., drowning out the incessant traffic noise three floors below. The last number finally answered, the woman an actress, her voice Shakespearean, totally unlike the Lisa Waters Jennifer had met. Frustrated, she folded out her sleep-sofa and decided to wash her hair before bed.

Jennifer slipped off her robe and set the shampoo and bath towel beside the kitchen sink. A fingernail tap on the goldfish bowl brought Sushi and Saki face to face with her as she adjusted the water temperature just the way she liked it for her shampoo. "No treats tonight," she told them. "You're getting fat."

The sink basin was the perfect depth to get her head under the faucet, the cabinet was the right height to bend over without strain, and the warm water pummeled and soothed her scalp and tense neck muscles. Rising steam opened her nostrils and lubricated her throat, dry from fruitless conversation. She shampooed her long hair leisurely, rinsing and lathering again. Her breath caught for an instant when she thought she heard something bump against the apartment door. She listened intently, raising her dripping head from the sink, the only sound a loud hissing as the faucet sprayed water into the sink. She wiped soap from one eye and surveyed the room behind her. Only Sushi and Saki were there, unblinking, watching her every move. "David?" she called, instinctively covering her bare breasts with her arms. No answer. She called again, heard nothing above the roar of the water. "Getting paranoid," she told her fish, and doused her head back under the faucet. Water ran across her face, into her ears, around her neck as she rinsed her hair again, muffling all sound. She reached blindly for the shampoo bottle once more just as an icy draft chilled the back of her neck and something grabbed her from behind. She stifled a scream, dropped the shampoo as a strong hand encircled her neck. "David," she tried to yell, choking, her heart suddenly in her throat, and furious at his game. She hit the back of her head painfully when she jerked her head up, but was instantly plunged back into the foaming sink, her cheek smacking against the side. Powerful hands clutched at her head despite her efforts to free herself, and she vaguely felt the shampoo bottle squirt out from beneath one foot. She screamed a desperate but muffled cry as her feet flew out from under her in the greasy goo, and struck her chest a hard blow against the countertop, her arms useless and weak against a greater strength. She kicked painfully against something hard and unyielding as she thrashed about, struggling frantically for air, dimly aware of a shattering sound somewhere nearby. Water filled her ears and clogged her stinging nostrils. The faucet's spray hammered at her skull like hail on a coffin, all light blotted out from her straining eyes. Gasping sobs and muffled cries clotted in her throat as hot fragrant water rose to cover her head, blotting out all sound except the internal gurgle that strangled and seared her fiery lungs.

9

———◦━━◆━━◦———

Jennifer coughed, gagged, and expelled a slimy rush of soapy water onto the rug on which she lay. When she lifted her head, the ceiling spun dizzyingly above her, an amorphous face floating somewhere between. Sounds began to reenter her consciousness as she gasped for air and tried to focus her eyes.

"You all right, doctor?" a distant voice echoed.

The face of the balding building superintendent slowly emerged from the amorphous blob suspended over her. Jennifer tried to speak, grabbed at her screaming ribs as a spasm of coughing racked her body, and almost blacked out again. She turned on her side, sputtered and hacked, bubbly water gushing from her nose and mouth. At last she saw the colors of the rug, an arm, a hand. Hers. And she knew she was alive. Suddenly shaking with cold, she pulled something around her neck and sat up, wondering how the towel got draped over her naked body. As her mind cleared, she froze in disbelief, as though an icy hand had encircled her heart. "Sushi," she screamed. "Saki." She lunged forward with abandon, ignoring the bits of shattered glass on the floor, quickly scooping the still gold bodies of her fish into her palms.

"Too late," the super said. "They's dead when I got here."

Ignoring his remark, Jennifer held their limp little bodies under the tap with one hand while she hurriedly grabbed and filled a soup bowl with the other. Straining to will them to live, gently pressing and releasing their sides alternately with her fingers in hopes of resuscitating them, she slipped to the floor on her knees as first Sushi, then Saki slowly floated to the top of the water on their sides, their lustrous golden tails trailing motionless behind. "Oh, God, no," she groaned, her head falling to her chest, her body racked with sobs.

It was some time later when Jennifer was able to put on her robe and slippers and hold a cup of tea on her lap while the superintendent told her what he'd found.

"Came to change the bulb in the hall outside after Mrs. Brant complained, and heard something banging and thrashing inside your place. I knocked on the door, called out, and when you didn't answer, I forced the door open. The window there was up, and I found you like a half-drowned puppy on the floor. I figured you fell, maybe hit your head."

Jennifer coughed into a handkerchief, blew her stinging nose. "Did you see him?" she rasped.

The super shook his head. "I didn't see nobody."

"He tried to kill me." The realization was awesome, unreal. "And he killed my fish." Jennifer picked up the phone, dialed the operator, asked for the police. While she waited, the super went downstairs to tell his wife, then came back, a can of beer in hand.

Twenty minutes later, two policemen arrived, quickly checked the tiny apartment, the fire escape, the alley below. They found nothing.

"Light bulb in the hall's unscrewed. He must have gone down the fire escape," the ruddy-faced senior officer said. "Any idea who'd want to kill you? Maybe scare you?"

Jennifer shook her head, twisted at her handkerchief, her throat raw and scratchy.

The officer looked out her window again into the sleeting night. "Have you enticed anybody, teased them?"

She didn't understand.

"You know, undress in front of the open window? Walk around nude?" He turned to face her.

"What kind of question is that?" she demanded.

"Depends," he said. "What kind of person are you? We see all sorts."

Furious but still frightened, Jennifer quickly realized the cops would do nothing to catch the intruder. They said they'd file a report, suggested she put a better lock on her door. Maybe bar the windows. They left.

Jennifer turned to thank the balding superintendent, watched his gaze slowly fall to her breasts and rise again. She folded her arms, thanked him again for coming to her rescue, and said good night.

It was nearly dawn when Jennifer fell asleep, her desk wedged against the front door, all her lights burning brightly. She hoped there really was a giant goldfish bowl somewhere above the sky.

Jennifer awakened a little after ten Saturday morning, feeling as though she had gone ten rounds with Kid Foster. Every muscle ached, her ribs were sore, her neck stiff, her throat raspy and thick. There were bruises on her arms, her thighs, a scab on the instep of one foot. Bloodshot brown eyes stared back from her bathroom mirror, her tangled hair a reminder of her terror the night before. The memory made her shudder.

Almost instinctively she caught herself starting for the goldfish food after brushing her teeth. Reluctantly she dropped the plastic bag of pellets into the trash.

Before lunch, Jennifer walked to Bloomingdale's, never before fully appreciating the beauty of such a crisp, bright January day. Scattered patches of shadowed ice melted along the sidewalks where the sun hadn't yet found them, and the cold sky was summer-blue and clear. She selected a blue velour zipper-bag sleep outfit and doggie rattle for Juan Ortez from the infants' department, browsed women's coats and jeans, and went back outside on Third Avenue to just appreciate being alive. A light lunch at Yellowfingers, people-watching, then a brisk walk home.

She kept on her jeans and alpaca sweater when she went to deliver her present to Maria. Even Mrs. Rogers, former nurse, couldn't ban her from the hospital as a visitor.

"Gone," the floor nurse said. "Just disappeared. Before the morning shift came on. Her baby, too."

Jennifer had half-expected Maria to be gone, but she had to be sure. The aide in the nursery confirmed the report.

Jennifer stood at Melanie's bedside in silence for a long while, trying to understand what had made the spunky young woman break. Still staked out at all four corners, bound and gagged, Melanie thrashed and struggled desperately against private devils in her own hell. A pretty black private-duty nurse passed on the psychiatrist's opinions. She was sympathetic and attentive, but her eyes held little hope for Melanie's future. Intravenous fluids dripped silently and steadily into Melanie's veins, providing nourishment and fluids, while regular injections of tranquilizers did little to give her rest. Jennifer helped the nurse shift and work around Melanie to change the bed when an involuntary bowel movement suddenly soiled her sheets.

Jennifer asked if Melanie's relatives had been notified. The nurse lowered her eyes. "She has none." Her long lashes blinked, raised. "Her roommate was here earlier. She brought flowers." She indicated an arrangement of red and white carnations beside the bed.

Jennifer finally said good-bye, slowly walked once around the block, and went home. Her depression lifted for a while after she spoke with Maria on the phone.

"My son, he es happy. He love it at home."

Jennifer said she had a gift for Juan. She'd try to bring it by within the week.

"I comin' to the baby doctor," Maria said. "I see you then. Next week."

After she hung up, Jennifer washed out her underclothes and hung them to dry on the shower-curtain rod. She ate an early dinner alone, barricaded her door with her desk, and fell asleep by ten P.M.

It was nearly midnight when Maria Ortez gently removed her full brown nipple from her son's mouth, pressed him to her shoulder, and patted until he burped, went back to sleep. She laid him in the padded wooden box beside her bed, careful to support his heavy head, and tucked the new blanket around the sides. Climbing into her own narrow bed, she turned off the lamp and held her breath, listening, to make sure he was breathing all right. Something scratched against the wall across the darkened room, scurried off before she could reach the light. Little Juan kicked once in his sleep, moved his lips, and then was still. Maria tried to ignore the drunken shouts from the bar downstairs, pulled the covers around her cold neck, and went to sleep, facing her son.

Nurse Kane arrived at the clinic less than a half-hour after Josef's call Sunday morning. She walked quickly down the corridor past the lab, unlocked a door, entered a narrow gray hallway with closed metal doors on either side. Josef opened the last door just before she reached it. Weak, moaning sobs came from within. Kane marched straight past Josef to Laniet Teague's bedside and turned. Josef stepped inside and closed the door. "When?" Kane demanded.

"Found her that way this morning. You can't even touch her."

Kane reached for Laniet's arm, barely made contact with her skin. Laniet recoiled violently, shrieked a bloodcurdling scream piercing enough to chill the ghosts of the nearby morgue. Kane stood rigid, watched as the flushed red-headed girl dissolved into gasping sobs. "What hurts?" Kane asked.

Laniet Teague tried to speak, her breath catching. Kane turned to stare at Josef. "Did you do anything to her, Josef?"

He shook his head and leaned back against the door. "No."

"Don't lie to me, Josef."

"I'm not that way anymore, Nurse Kane. Honest." His basso rumble echoed in the concrete room.

Kane turned back to Laniet. "What hurts? Did Josef hurt you?"

Laniet tried to shake her head, winced, her eyes squeezed tightly shut. "Everything. Arm, toe, skin. Everything." She lay perfectly still, as though afraid to move.

Kane walked past the wooden chair to the pain-control console across the room, opened the notebook. "Thirty-four was her highest pain tolerance?"

Josef didn't move from the door, but nodded.

Kane took a deep breath. "That was last night?"

He nodded again. "Then she passed out, like always."

Kane removed her black overcoat, folded it on the console desk. "The medicine finally wore off. Put her in the chair, Josef."

Laniet shouted, screamed, cried, and begged as Josef untied her and strapped her into the heavy wooden test chair. The lightest touch seemed to cause extreme agony. She swore that merely applying the adhesive-backed wires to her fingers was excruciating.

Kane ignored her pleas, turned on the machine. At a dial setting midway between 0 and 1, Laniet's eyes seemed to bulge, the veins in her neck and forehead at bursting capacity, her skin blotched, irregular. A pathetic animal sound came from somewhere deep in her throat. Kane raised the dial to level 1.

"Please," Laniet wailed. "No more."

Laniet lost consciousness at pain level 3, puddles of sweat spreading out around her bare feet. Kane made several notes, stood, and left the room.

In the computer room, Nurse Kane pressed the keys for number 997, glanced at the readout, erased that portion of the tape, and switched the computer off. She went to the clinic, opened the medication cabinet, and poured seven cc's of Opain into a paper cup, adding water from the tap. Josef was tightening the bed's strap around Laniet's wrist below her cast when Kane reentered the unconscious girl's room. "Josef," she chastised, pulling the white hospital gown down over the exposed red triangle of hair between Laniet's porcelain legs. Josef grumbled something deep under his breath, left the room.

Minutes later, Laniet began to groan, then opened her questioning eyes, disoriented. Kane held the cup to the girl's parched lips. "Drink this." She did, her expression more one of desperate fear than trust.

Kane walked out to where Josef waited in the hall. "Test her again this evening. How's the other one? Lisa Waters."

Josef stared down at Nurse Kane for a long moment. "Up to eighteen. But she's not as strong as this one. I thought her heart had stopped this morning."

Kane narrowed her eyes. "What was her blood pressure?"

"One-seventy over one-ten."

"Pulse?"

"One-eighty-five."

Kane pulled on her coat, tied her scarf, turned to leave. "She'll be all right."

At six Sunday evening, Jennifer Barton folded her checkbook and tossed it on top of the New York *Times* on her desk. No matter how many times she subtracted the numbers, she had two-hundred eighty-four dollars and change to her name. She picked up the phone on its first ring, suddenly aware of the frustration her own voice conveyed.

"You don't sound very happy. How about that dinner I promised you?"

"Dr. Neilson. Boy, am I glad to talk to you."

Jennifer agreed to be in front of her apartment building at seven. Neilson pulled his sleek silver Mercedes up a few minutes early, but Jennifer was ready. She'd decided on her brown wool sweater and skirt, brown pumps. In the car, she started to tell Neilson about Melanie Wardner.

"Huh-uh," he said. "Not tonight. That's business. This is strictly pleasure."

In his apartment, Jennifer sipped a glass of white Lillet and watched, amazed, as Neilson prepared *coq au vin*. A crackling fire in the fireplace took her back to her childhood, even smelled the same. Burning oak. Like when her aunt came to visit for Thanksgiving, and her mother fixed a turkey with all the trimmings. She loved Neilson's apartment. It was velvety soft, in burgundies, but masculine. One entire wall was solid books. From the dining-alcove window she could see three different bridges, their lights twinkling like tiny stars over the East River, twenty stories below.

Jennifer waited till after their elegant dinner before mentioning her job. Neilson blew out the candles on the dining table, brought Jennifer a cup of coffee, and joined her on the couch before the fire.

"I forgot all about that," he said. "Forgive me. I'll go by Rogers' office first thing tomorrow." He asked for details of why she was suspended. He listened patiently, frowned. "I think you behaved admirably. Every man has a right to die the way he wants to. And without pain. Mr. Jackson found solace in his whiskey and his cigarettes. He tried to soothe his pains the only way he knew." Neilson patted Jennifer's hand. "Consider yourself reinstated. If they object, or drag it out, I'll hire you as my personal assistant."

Jennifer thanked him. His blue eyes were intent, sincere, reflections of the fire's yellow flames dancing in them. "I couldn't ask you to do that," she said.

"Nonsense. What do they pay you?"

"Twelve hundred a month."

Neilson laughed. "I pay Josef more than that. All right. Until this is settled, you're on my payroll. Two thousand a month. Okay?"

She shook her head, toyed with the weight of the coffee cup in her hand. "It's not the money. I've got to get that fellowship."

Neilson asked why it was so important to her.

"I love reconstructive surgery," she said. "To put people back together after accidents. After mutilating cancer surgery." She looked up into his face. "I'm pretty good at it now. But I need the extra training. I want to be the best."

"Do you have a job waiting? A practice?"

She nodded. "In Atlanta. I'm joining a group of head-and-neck surgeons. But they need somebody July 1, for coverage. If I don't get my fellowship soon, they'll take somebody else."

"You'll get it," he said.

Later, Dr. Neilson set two tulip-shaped glasses on the coffee table and brought out a bottle of champagne. Dom Perignon. "A celebration," he said, popping the cork against the ceiling.

Jennifer could see the excitement in his eyes. "What is it?" she asked. "Tell me."

He touched his glass to hers. "To eradicating pain and suffering from this earth," he said. "Opain works." He grinned like a little boy with a new red bicycle.

"You tabulated the results? The study?"

He nodded, beaming with delight, and they drank the toast.

"It's perfect," he said. "Absolute pain relief with no sedation, no addiction, no respiratory depression. Think of it. In the future, there'll be no need for other pain medications. Aspirin, morphine, codeine. All of them obsolete."

Jennifer wanted to hug him. "When?" she said. "How long before it's released?"

His eyes changed slightly. "In some parts of the world, within weeks."

She asked him to explain. "The FDA requires years of testing," she said.

Neilson sat closer beside her, stared at the fire. "They may have to change their regulations this time." He finished his glass of champagne, poured another. "Did you know there's an enzyme available in Europe that completely dissolves herniated disks with one injection?"

"No."

"Most Americans don't. They've proven its use in Europe for over twelve years. The FDA won't release it in the States. Since the Thalidomide incident, the rest of the world has treatments for cancer, heart medications, blood-pressure drugs, steroids—the list is endless—that our patients can't get. We live in the most affluent, most advanced country in the world. And our people suffer, some totally incapacitated, because of a federal government that has grown too large, too powerful. I will not allow that to happen with Opain."

Jennifer heard his voice break with emotion, saw the moisture fill his eyes. "How can you avoid it?" she asked.

He raised his eyebrows, studied his glass, then smiled. "I already have." He turned to look at her. "Within weeks, the FDA will beg me to release Opain in the United States. The citizens will be in the streets, outraged, until they do." He smiled again, set his glass down, traced a line on Jennifer's cheek with his finger, touched her lip. "That's what we celebrate tonight."

Jennifer saw the satisfaction in his eyes. Sensed the power he felt. "You sold the formula," she said.

He lowered his face close to hers, made a low, throaty sound, almost a chuckle. "Never," he whispered. "Every single vial will be bought from me."

His lips were soft and warm on hers, tender at first, then more demanding. She heard his breathing change, drew back just enough to see his face, the question in his eyes. "Congratulations," she said. She touched a finger to the tip of his nose. "I know it's trite, but it is getting late. Drive me home?"

Without moving, he asked, "Have you ever made love to a multibillionaire?"

She grinned. "No. Have you?"

Neilson laughed, took her hand, and stood. "Come to think of it, I haven't. At least, not yet."

On the drive home, Jennifer asked, "What would you do if the government could stop Opain? Maybe took it away from you?"

Neilson's jaw set firmly, but he answered immediately. "Start over," he said. "In another country."

Jennifer thought for a moment. "But they'd have the formula. How could you compete?"

"It's a very tricky formula," he said. "A tiny substitution on a tyrosine amino acid. Only Nurse Kane and I know exactly how it's done."

"But a good lab man could analyze it. Duplicate it."

"Maybe. But I have worldwide patents this time. To protect it."

Back in her tiny apartment, Jennifer sat at her desk and wrote:

Dear Steve,
   I sure could use some of your advice and wisdom right now. Things are happening so fast I am thoroughly confused. Most of all, I would like to feel you beside me again. To just know you were there. Then the other things wouldn't matter quite so much. I love you, my darling. I always will.

A tear spilled over onto one corner of the blue stationery as Jennifer folded it carefully. She dabbed at her eye, dropped the letter into the wastebasket, went to bed.

In her second-floor flat near Bedford-Stuyvesant, Maria Ortez slept soundly, huddled under a thin blanket beside the homemade bassinet that cradled her son. The usual shouting and fighting noises outside had ended hours earlier, when the bar closed and the drunks finally dispersed throughout the cold city. Little Juan kicked at his blankets again, one bare foot scraping against the wooden interior of his bed. The scratching noise behind the wall stopped for a moment; then fast little toenails, ticking like jacks dropped on plastic, scurried across the cheap linoleum floor. Juan kicked again, freeing his foot from the blue blanket, and abraded the skin of his big

toe, drops of bright red blood trickling into the spaces
between his toes and down his restless foot. He made a
soft cooing noise. Moments later, something long and
brown leaped silently from the bedside table into the
baby's bassinet, causing him to jump, as if startled, but
purely by reflex. Maria was awakened some twenty
minutes later by a strange gnawing sound, like the sharp
teeth of a puppy trying to eat a beef bone. She turned
on the bedside lamp, screamed to wake the living dead
and everybody else in her building. She jumped frantically out of bed, swatting at a scruffy brown rat resting
back on its blood-smeared haunches gnawing at the
bloody bone stub of her baby's big toe. She had to hold
to the edge of the table to keep from fainting. The rat
scampered over the top of the bassinet-box, jumped to
the linoleum floor, and darted across the room under a
sagging overstuffed chair, a piece of bloody brown flesh
and fragment of tiny toenail protruding from one side of
its slim and grinning jaws. Little Juan sucked furiously
and happily at his thin brown lips.

10

Jennifer got up early Monday morning, ironed her white uniform jacket, smoothed her shoulder-length brown hair in the bathroom mirror, and decided against wearing lipstick to the medical-board hearing. When she arrived at the medical-staff office ten minutes early, she was instructed to take a seat outside the meeting room and wait. It was almost eight-thirty when she was asked inside.

Twelve distinguished and concerned faces studied her as she took the empty seat facing their long table. Half-filled coffee cups and water glasses sat beside lined yellow legal tablets in front of the physicians. Dr. Yardley, chief of the department of medicine, nodded toward Nurse Rogers, turned to Jennifer. "You're aware of the charges against you, Dr. Barton?"

Jennifer tried to moisten her lips with a sandpaper tongue. "Yes."

Neither Yardley's face nor his voice gave any suggestion of emotion. "Please tell us exactly what happened with this patient, Mr. Jackson, in the emergency room."

Jennifer related her experience, attempting to be factual and objective. She brushed a tear from one cheek as she finished. When she stopped, nobody spoke. One physician stared at the ceiling, hands intertwined behind his hairless head; another concentrated on the point where he tapped his yellow pencil on his notepad. Somebody coughed and shuffled his feet. Mrs. Rogers pursed her prim little mouth and stared somewhere beyond Jennifer's shoulder.

"If you'll wait outside," Dr. Yardley said, "we'll discuss your case."

Jennifer returned to the uncomfortable chair in the waiting room, tried to thumb through old issues of *National Geographic*. She wondered what Nurse Rogers was saying about her. The acne-scarred emergency-room nurse avoided Jennifer's eyes when she entered, was quickly admitted to the hearing room. She glanced sheepishly toward Jennifer when she exited several minutes later. Jennifer wondered if Dr. Neilson had already come by, or if he had forgotten about her again.

After what seemed an eternity she was called back inside. Jennifer wiped her damp palms on her skirt, forced her chin high, and entered on unsteady legs.

". . . one week's suspension," Yardley was saying. "The Head and Neck service concurs that there was no way to save the man's life. And you did ask for an emergency consult." Yardley cleared his throat, lowered his bushy eyebrows. "There is no excuse, however, for breaking the regulations about smoking and drinking in the hospital." He paused. "Dr. Neilson has agreed to employ you during your suspension, as his associate. One week from today, you go back on the hospital payroll. You may stay in Brigton House, meanwhile."

Jennifer wanted to jump in the air and shout. They'd found her innocent of any wrongdoing. The mild slap on the wrists was obviously to mollify Rogers. She respectfully said, "Yes, sir."

"But let me caution you," Yardley added. "Familiarize yourself with hospital regulations. Another offense and you'll be dismissed. Is that clear?"

She felt her relief wane. "Yes, sir."

He punctuated his final words with a nod. "You may go, doctor."

In the pain clinic that morning Nurse Kane was no

more distant than usual, shuffled patients in and out as always. Jennifer took an immediate liking to her third patient, Stephanie Adams.

"But everybody calls me Steph," the trim brunette said, smiling. "Anyway, Dr. Pearl, he's my dentist, says I'm the worst patient he's ever seen. I mean, I try, but I just can't stand the thought of having my teeth drilled into. You know? That little whiny-sounding drill? And I hate those shots they give you that paralyze your whole face numb so you can't drink anything all day long without it dribbling all over your chin."

Jennifer finally learned that Stephanie Adams was to have a root canal done in the next few days, and Dr. Pearl had requested a consult regarding her pain tolerance. On the threshold stimulator, Steph topped out at level 4. Within normal limits. Jennifer told her so, wished her good luck, and turned her over to Nurse Kane.

As Kane opened the medication room, Jennifer watched to see if she would select from box number three, Opain, for Stephanie. An unexpected whisper in Jennifer's ear and a touch on her hair caused her to jump. "Dr. Neilson," she exclaimed.

He grinned, beaming. "Congratulations," he said. "I just heard."

On impulse, Jennifer stretched up and kissed his cheek. "Thank you," she said. "For everything."

"Your next patient is waiting," Nurse Kane announced behind Jennifer.

Neilson seemed to stiffen, nodded to Jennifer, looked at Kane. "They only gave her a week's suspension," he said.

Without expression, Kane studied Neilson's face, turned, and walked away.

Just before lunch, Dr. Neilson knocked on Jennifer's examining-room door as she was finishing with her last patient of the morning. "Emergency consult from plastic surgery. Jennings, room 521. Sixty percent burns. I've got a TV interview to do, so check him out and give him this if he's not allergic to any medications." Neilson held out a filled syringe to her.

"What's in here?" she asked.

Neilson crinkled his eyes, smiled. "The same thing I'll be talking about on the TV show. Opain." He winked. "Try to watch it. They plan to repeat it on the six-o'clock news."

Jennifer had wanted to ask Neilson to go with her to see Melanie Wardner, but he'd already wheeled and left. She completed her patient's examination, left the chart with Nurse Kane, and went to the fifth floor.

A man's low, moaning sobs guided her to room 521. She put on a sterile gown, cap, and mask before entering the room, assisted by the man's private nurse. A gowned plastic-surgery resident hovered over the patient inside. "Hold still, dammit," the resident commanded.

The mummified man in bed yelled out an agonizing death cry that bombarded Jennifer's senses till she thought his lungs and her eardrums must surely burst. The resident shouted angrily again, rubbed something white and greasy on the man's right leg. What remained of the patient's skin was like parched leather dried and preserved in a desert sun, mingled with areas of pure black eschar, dead, like charcoal, and raw, bleeding meat. His face was splotched and bloody, all hair gone from where his eyebrows and lashes had been. One ear was crumpled and black, like a deflated plastic toy. A sickening sweet-burned smell like singed pork ribs hung in Jennifer's nostrils.

"I'm Dr. Barton," Jennifer said to the resident's back.

He spun around, medicine jar and wooden applicator in his gloved hands.

"Pain Control," Jennifer said. The nauseating stench of scorched flesh permeated her mask.

"Thank God you finally got here," the resident said. "This guy is driving us all nuts. He's impossible."

Mr. Jennings' constant low groaning was escalating, as though he never paused to breathe. Jennifer asked about his burns.

"Gasoline explosion. On his yacht. He's some kind of

big businessman. Thirty percent third-degree burns, full thickness skin loss." The resident used the wooden applicator to tap on the blackened hard areas of the man's arms, legs, feet, and chest, more like the synthetic Bakelite than flesh. "Twenty percent second-degree, here and here." He touched one blistered, peeling island on the man's forehead, causing thick yellow fluid to gush from a lemon-sized blister and dribble into the man's open eye. Another agonizing yell immediately filled the room. The resident glowered at the patient, turned to Jennifer. "If he'd just stop that goddamned yelling. You can't touch him." He turned to the patient. "You're acting like a two-year-old. You should be ashamed of yourself."

Jennifer stepped forward immediately, asked Mr. Jennings, "Are you allergic to any medicines?"

The resident rose to his full height and answered as the man sobbed uncontrollably, his entire body shaking so violently the bed squeaked in rhythm with his convulsive sobs. "No allergies," the resident proclaimed.

Jennifer turned sideways, slipped in between the resident and Mr. Jennings, took the syringe from her coat pocket. "This is going to sting," she said. "But it'll help your pain." She injected the Opain with one smooth, rapid motion. Jennings didn't seem to notice, continued to cry.

The private nurse had an alcohol sponge extended toward Jennifer when she turned, her eyes questioning that Jennifer had ignored the age-old routine of ineffectively swabbing the skin before an injection. The accepted ritual, like a tribal dance.

"Do you think any bugs could have lived through that fire?" Jennifer asked.

The nurse blinked twice rapidly. "But infection . . ."

Jennifer nodded. "I know. But isopropyl alcohol takes several minutes to work. It just pushes the bacteria around, stirs them up." She looked at the perspiring resident. "The other ten percent?"

He hesitated, narrowed his eyes. "First-degree," he said. "Mostly on his abdomen."

Jennifer returned the resident's challenging gaze. "Have you ever experienced real pain, doctor?"

His eyes darted toward the private nurse, back to Jennifer. "I've had the normal ones."

Jennifer felt her scalp move beneath her sterile cap. "Pray you never do," she said.

On the fourteenth floor, Jennifer was relieved to see that Melanie Wardner was no longer bound and gagged. Melanie was deathly pale, her pulse weak and thready, her eyes hollow and rimmed with dark circles. Somehow, she appeared to have shrunk since Jennifer first met her. She was either comatose or sleeping, no movement visible except the faint shallow excursions of her chest as she breathed.

"She's better," the soft voice of a pretty black nurse said as she stepped up to the side of the bed next to Jennifer.

Melanie's eyelids twitched, slowly opened. She turned her head toward Jennifer. Her voice was weak, distant, when she spoke. "Dr. Barton." She tried to smile.

Jennifer took her limp hand. "It's okay, Melanie. Rest now. I'll see you later."

Melanie nodded, drifted back to sleep.

The nurse walked out into the hall with Jennifer. "She's exhausted, poor thing."

Jennifer agreed. "What has Dr. Bevins said?"

"Almost nothing. He just comes in, looks at her, and shakes his head. Her bladder seems to be fine now."

Jennifer noticed the "No Visitors" sign on the door. "Does her roommate know she's better?"

"She came by with more flowers and a card. I let her peek in for a minute. The psychiatrist doesn't want her disturbed."

Jennifer nodded, said good-bye, started to leave. "You have my home number?"

The nurse said she did, and Jennifer left.

As Jennifer walked down the hall toward the hospital cafeteria, David West called out her name, came up behind her. "How about a hamburger?" he asked. "Up the street."

"I left my coat in the clinic. I'll freeze."

He laughed, took her arm. "We'll run."

Over a hamburger and Coke, Jennifer told David what she'd learned about his former patient Arnold Heath.

West scrunched up his eyes at the thought. "Jesus," he said. "What a way to go."

"The highway-patrol clerk said there was a witness. But he couldn't do anything to help. Said the expressway traffic was so heavy they just kept running over him, bouncing him along the pavement, and hitting him again."

West shook his head, grimaced. Neither spoke for a long moment. "David, did he know he had a brain tumor?"

West frowned, looked surprised. "Sure. I explained it to him. He had to know something was causing those headaches."

Jennifer tried to sort it out in her mind. "Maybe that explains it," she said. "He wanted to end it quickly, without the long suffering."

West set his glass on the table. Shook his head. "He wouldn't have suffered. His tumor was benign. Removable."

"You're sure?"

"Hey. I'm a neurosurgeon. Remember?"

"Did he know it was benign?"

"Of course. What are you getting at?"

Jennifer drew finger lines in the wet ring beside her glass on the wooden tabletop. "I'm not sure, David. I wish I knew."

West changed the subject, asked how she liked the surgery she'd seen. She complimented his work, said it had been fascinating, then abruptly asked, "Where were you Friday night?"

"Typical woman," he teased, grinning. "Buy you one hamburger and you get possessive."

She smiled, waited while he chewed.

"Southampton," he finally said. "Why?"

She sipped her Coke. "How did you know about Steve?"

"What is this, the Inquisition?" He sounded annoyed.

"I'd like to know."

West folded his napkin, turned over the check. "When I brought your purse and sweater to your apartment and you weren't there, I was looking for something to read while I waited. I tipped over the wastebasket, by accident, and saw a letter to Steve."

"And you read it?"

"No, I didn't. I just saw the name, put it back, and found Neilson's articles on the desk."

Jennifer tore little triangles from her paper napkin, twisted them, and dropped them in the ashtray. West paid the waiter, left a tip beside his plate, leaned forward on the table. "Jennie."

She looked up, saw his concerned face question her, a comma of coal-black hair on his forehead.

"What's wrong, Jennie?"

She took a deep breath, watched for his reaction. "Somebody tried to kill me Friday night. And they killed my goldfish."

In the lab that afternoon, Jennifer changed the subject every time David West brought up her attack. She'd told him everything she knew, admitted she had wondered about him, only because he had known how to get into her apartment so easily. "I don't want anybody else to know," she said. "It would look bad. I'm already suspended from the hospital."

"So who's here to listen?" West asked. "The animals?"

Jennifer lowered her voice. "Josef keeps coming in and out. You never know who's listening."

West laughed, whispered. "Now you're getting paranoid."

"Wouldn't you if somebody half-drowned you?"

"I'd get my lock changed." He hesitated. "Jennie, there have been several break-ins in staff housing. They're kids looking for drugs. You happened to be home, and the guy panicked."

"Maybe," she said.

"Look, I'll pick up a lock and install it for you. Okay?"

She shook her head. "I've already taken care of it. The super's going to put one in."

He took her hand for a moment. "Then no more talk about Nurse Kane hiding patients and people trying to murder you."

"Don't talk so loud," she whispered, pointing toward Josef, just going out the rear door.

West spoke in his normal tone. "Josef doesn't pay any attention to us. He's only interested in the animals. And whatever Nurse Kane says."

"He gives me the creeps."

West laughed again. "You watch too many horror movies. He's big and ugly, but he's not as dumb as he looks. Peculiar, maybe. Not dumb."

Jennifer disagreed.

"I saw him break down the pain-threshold machine one day," West said, "when it went on the blink during clinic. He took the circuit board apart, fixed it, and had it back together in no time. Even with Kane standing over him, bitching."

"He does jump when she says jump," Jennifer said.

The rear door opened just then, and Josef came into the lab. They forced their attention back to the experiment at hand, a pain-tolerance test on a guinea pig. The unknown drug being tested was working very poorly.

"Do you remember Lisa Waters?" Jennifer asked.

"No."

"Laniet Teague?"

"Should I?"

Jennifer shrugged. "I guess not. I just hoped maybe you'd seen them."

At five-thirty, Jennifer left the lab, checked on Melanie Wardner—condition unchanged, according to the blue-haired nurse she had met earlier—and raced across First Avenue toward David West's apartment to watch Dr. Neilson on color TV.

West answered the door in corduroy jeans and a blue sweater. Inside, Jennifer saw an English oak dining table littered with books and a human skull, only two oak chairs, and an incongruous vinyl sofa behind a round oak coffee table.

"That's next on my replacement list," West said, indicating the vinyl sofa.

"You like antiques," Jennifer observed.

He nodded, smiling. "They don't self-destruct like the new stuff."

She walked around the room admiring the feeling. It wasn't great decorating, but was somehow warm. Lived-in. She stopped at two framed photos on the far wall. One appeared to be a college graduation class, another was a football team. "You're an athlete?"

"Football and track," he said. "Ohio State."

She walked to a glass-front oak bookshelf, saw the trophies almost hidden inside. "You must have been pretty good."

"I enjoyed it," he said. "It was a good team."

She turned to study him. "Is that how you got through college? A football scholarship?"

He nodded. "That and tending bar at the local hangout."

"That doesn't leave much time for studying." Or girls, she thought.

"You manage," he said. "If you really want something."

Jennifer touched the surface of the oak table as she walked by, paused to trace her finger over pencil lines drawn on the back of the skull, obviously used to rehearse new surgical procedures. As she turned the skull around to face her, she laughed out loud. "He has a mustache," she said, brushing the backs of her fingers along a ridiculous handlebar mustache cemented above the exposed upper teeth. "What's his name?"

West grinned and came up beside her. "Count Mario DeVecchio. Notice the sheepish grin?"

She did.

"He's a famous fifteenth-century physician who declared that every possible major medical discovery had already been made. I keep him around to remind myself there may be better ways of doing things." West glanced at his watch and switched on the TV.

On the six-o'clock news, after Neilson was introduced and his long list of credentials mentioned by the newscaster, Neilson's opening line was, "I have discovered the perfect pain reliever."

11

---❖——❖————❖———

Jennifer was shocked at Neilson's blatant statement. He'd always seemed so professional. Almost retiring.

"Well, it's true," West said. "He's been too cautious in his earlier interviews. Now he's going for broke." Jennifer hunched forward on West's sofa.

". . . a drug which will relieve every type pain, from the most minor scratchy throat to the most severe pains imaginable," Neilson said. "Burns, renal colic from kidney stones, migraine headaches, the unrelenting chronic pains of arthritis, degenerated spines, cancer, broken hips."

"Isn't that rather a broad claim, doctor?"

Neilson stared directly into the camera, his face serious, unblinking. "It is a statement of fact. I have the experiments to back it up. Tests in thousands of laboratory animals. Over a thousand human patients."

"Is it habit-forming?" the reporter asked, his voice challenging, doubtful.

"There are no bad side effects," Neilson calmly said.

The reporter looked amused. "And where can we get this wonder drug, doctor? What do you call it?"

"It's called Opain," Neilson said. "And it isn't available."

The reporter asked him to explain.

"I am about to enter into an agreement with a multinational pharmaceutical company for Opain to be released in a foreign country, after they confirm its effectiveness. In fact, they have supported my work through donations, eliminating the need for government grants."

"Yet you say this panacea—this cure for all ills—is not available here. Surely it will be, if it can do what you claim."

"Opain doesn't cure anything except pain. But it absolutely eliminates any need for pain or suffering from any known disease. It will not be available to United States citizens, however."

"Do you have something against us, doctor?" The reporter flashed a plastic smile.

"No. I love my country. But the United States government, through its Food and Drug Administration, the FDA, requires years of testing and millions of dollars of expenditures before a new drug can be sold in this country."

"Dr. Neilson," the perfect voice said, "as we all know, there are many, many painkilling drugs on the market today. Hundreds over-the-counter. Others by prescription. These drugs are tried and tested, known to be effective. What prompted you to announce your new drug now? When it isn't yet available? And why should we believe there's even a need for it?"

Neilson turned to the sanctimonious reporter, nodded toward the phone on his desk. "Ask the switchboard to open up your phone lines. Give the station's phone number over the air, and ask only those people who are suffering right now—people in pain who are not relieved by the medicines they've been given—to call."

The reporter ignored the challenge. "Doctor, I'm afraid we're out of time. But thank you." The camera zoomed in on his dramatic face. "We have been talking to Dr. Franklyn Neilson of the Pain Control Clinic at . . ."

"Whew," West declared. "That's strong."

Jennifer sat back, watched him turn off the set. "He's absolutely right, you know. There must be millions of people out there hurting right now. I just hope he's right about no bad side effects."

"Such as?"

"I don't know. I'd love to ask him. Or see the results of the study on the computer." She watched as West opened a bottle of wine, poured two glasses. "You remember that rat that went nuts? Bashed his head against the cage?"

West raised his glass to her in a toast, tasted his wine. "It'd be hard to forget." He sat beside her.

"What if he wasn't 'cage-crazy,' as Josef called it? What if that was a reaction to Opain?"

West smiled his white smile. "Then Neilson would know. He's got access to the records, the computer tapes. He wouldn't lie about something like that."

Jennifer sipped her wine, set it down unfinished. "I'm sure you're right. It's much too important to him." She stood to leave.

"I thought you might stay awhile. We can send out for pizza or Chinese." West reached for her hand, caressed her fingers in his.

"Not tonight, David. I've got calls to make and some reading I must do."

West stood, lifted her chin, and searched her eyes. "Still Steve?" he asked.

She took a deep breath, kissed him on the cheek. "Good night, David. Thanks for the wine."

At home, Jennifer called to check on Ella Lu Mavis.

"Seem to be fine," her mother said in her gospel voice.

"No more pain? She acting all right?"

"I reckon. She been watchin' the TV all day."

"Could I speak with her?" Jennifer asked.

"If she was here. She gone out somewhere. Said she'd be back early, but she won't. That child love to stay out in the night."

Jennifer hung up, tried Maria Ortez's number, got no answer. She heated a can of vegetable-beef soup, ate while she read her current AMA *Journal*, and changed into her robe and slippers. At nine P.M. she moved her desk against the front door, filled the tub with hot water, and undressed for a bath. Her bruises were beginning to turn yellow around the edges, a good sign. The scrape on her foot was clean and dry. She was about to step into the tub when the phone rang; she grabbed her robe and ran through the open bathroom door to answer it.

". . . come over for a nightcap," Dr. Neilson said. "I'll pick you up in fifteen minutes." His voice was smooth and sensual, but his words slow, almost slurred.

"Have you been drinking?" she asked, laughing.

"A little. And why not? Did you see the show?"

She said she had. "You were very good."

Neilson laughed. "Wait till tomorrow. The A.M. show, *Good Morning America. The Tonight Show*'s called already."

Jennifer sat on the arm of her chair. "You're kidding."

Neilson didn't answer right away. She heard him swallow. "Every TV station's phone lines lit up like Rockefeller Plaza at Christmas," he said. "They couldn't handle the calls."

"People in pain?"

"You got it. Come on over, I'll tell you about it."

"I can't. Really. I was just getting into the tub."

He whistled softly. "There's a tub over here."

"Thanks anyway, mine's already filled. Besides, you'd better get some sleep. Sounds like you've got a busy schedule ahead."

"Maybe tomorrow, then. I'll take the phone off the hook so we won't be disturbed. It's been ringing all night."

"Maybe," she said. "And, congratulations." She hung up, removed her robe, and sat backward to soak in her hot tub so she could watch the living-room door, then went to bed.

The next morning, Jennifer put on her London Fog coat and a scarf and walked leisurely along First Avenue to the hospital, enjoying the crisp air. Fat, dark-bottomed clouds above the towering main building of the university hospital held a definite promise of snow. On the fourteenth floor Melanie Wardner still looked pale and drained, but smiled weakly and acknowledged Jennifer's visit. The floor nurse said Melanie had eaten a little custard at breakfast. Her private-duty day nurse had been canceled.

On the fifth floor, her burn patient, Mr. Jennings, seemed greatly improved. Jennifer had to lean close to understand what he said, since his face was covered with a heavy, stiff scab and his mouth hardly moved.

"Stiff," he managed. "No hurt."

"No pain? None at all?"

He barely nodded, blinked the eye that wasn't stuck together by a heavy yellowish-brown crust. As Jennifer turned to leave, Jennings suffered a spasm of coughing, spit up a thick ropy phlegm tinged with blood. She carefully wiped it from his raw chin with a tissue.

He blinked his eye. "Thank you."

In the hall outside, the plastic-surgery resident stopped Jennifer. "What was in that shot you gave Jennings?"

She hesitated. "I don't think I can say. It's Dr. Neilson's drug."

"Opain?"

"How did you know?"

He cocked his curly head to one side. "Honey, everybody in the city knows about Neilson's wonder drug. Don't you watch television?"

Jennifer said she had seen his interview.

The resident visually checked her figure, winked. "If he needs a testimonial, you let me know. Jennings hasn't made a whimper since you gave him that shot. Even when we put on his burn cream. I'll have him in the hydrotherapy tub by tomorrow."

Jennifer made a note in Mr. Jennings' chart and headed for the clinic. She was not prepared, however, for what she found there. The entire hallway leading from the elevators to the pain clinic was jammed with pushing, shoving people. Angry voices shouted unintelligibly above the din, and one elderly woman on crutches was pushed off balance by a sweaty-faced fat man who almost trampled her as he forced his way into the crowd beyond. Jennifer helped lift the old woman to her feet, unable to hear what she said.

"It's a doctor," somebody shouted behind Jennifer. "Let us through." A well-dressed graying man with ruddy cheeks grabbed Jennifer's arm and propelled her forward through the tangle of straining bodies. "Doctor," he shouted. "Let us through." Hostile faces softened instantly as people recognized Jennifer's white uniform, the man using her as a wedge to open an erratic path through the pulsating mob. A blustering, wide-eyed uniformed guard caught in the midst of the crowd helped separate tightly packed bodies ahead of Jennifer and the man who pushed from the rear, the crowd opening momentarily, then instantly closing ranks behind, swallowing them up. Hordes of anxious people filled the spaces around and behind the reception desk, and pounded on the closed doors to the examination rooms and animal lab. Jennifer suddenly felt trapped, enclosed, too tightly surrounded, and struggled to get more air in her lungs. Compressed in the crowd, a flash of heat surged through her, and she thought she would surely choke on the stale air. She felt the blood drain from her head as she pounded on the door to the lab and shouted her name above the deafening roar. The door opened a tiny crack, and Josef pulled her inside by one arm, using the full force of his body to close the door against the man behind her as she slipped through.

Jennifer almost collapsed onto a stool, stripping off her coat and loosening her scarf. "Where's Dr. Neilson?"

Josef stood against the door. "Not here."

"He's doing another TV show," Nurse Kane said, walking forward from the back of the room.

"What's going on out there?" Jennifer asked.

Kane almost smiled, but only with her mouth. "The people are demanding Opain. Dr. Neilson's drug."

"They've gone mad," Jennifer declared. "Like animals."

Kane narrowed her eyes. "It's only begun." She picked up the phone, dialed a number, asked for the producer of the evening news. "I'd suggest you get a re-

porter and cameraman over here right away," Kane said.
She repeated the call to several TV stations and the New
York *Times*.

People outside continued to bang on or bump against
the locked door, often shouting for Opain, giving Jennifer the uncomfortable feeling of being in a flimsy
small-town jail with a lynch mob outside. Nurse Kane
calmly set a portable TV on the countertop and
switched it on. She turned the dials until she found what
she wanted. The scene was along First Avenue, outside
New Hope University Hospital, with traffic at a blaring
standstill as throngs of people spilled over into the streets
from the hospital entrances and sidewalks. A young
brunette newswoman with one eye off-center shouted
above the noise about the incredible response to Dr.
Franklyn Neilson's announcement of his perfect painkiller, Opain. Mounted policemen attempted to herd the
people back onto the sidewalks as a distant bullhorn am-
plified orders to break it up and go home. The scene was
like an antiwar demonstration Jennifer had seen on TV
years before, but the faces in the crowd were mostly
older, strained, but equally concerned. The camera focused on a hand-lettered placard which read "FDA—NO,"
then another, "DOWN WITH PAIN."

Midway through the newscast, Nurse Kane turned
from the screen to Josef. "I believe you have work to
do," she said.

Josef turned and left through the rear door from the
animal lab.

It was nearly noon when police officers finally cleared
the clinic's reception area and hallway. Jennifer emerged
to see no-nonsense officers standing side by side, uniformed and helmeted, nightsticks at the ready, in front
of the rope barricades. The reception counter leaned
precariously against the gray wall near the clinic entrance, and the door to the medication room appeared
battered but intact.

Nurse Kane spoke from behind Jennifer. "We'll have
to move the records and medications to the rear. They'll
be back." She wheeled and walked toward the lab.

Jennifer slipped on her coat, put the scarf in her coat pocket, and began picking up battered pencils, paper clips, a trampled calendar, and the mangled, shoe-imprinted patient questionnaires that had spilled from the desktop to the floor. She stopped short when she saw the open bottom drawer behind the distorted counter-desk. Kane was nowhere in sight. Jennifer quickly extracted the heavy appointment book, tore out the pages from December 1 to the present, stuffed them in her coat pocket, and replaced the book. As a second thought, she pulled two other appointment books free, ripped out pages at random, and scattered them on the floor beneath the desk, along with the books themselves. Hearing the back door to the lab slam, she busied herself on the other side of the reception area, righting overturned wooden benches as Kane and Josef approached.

Kane concentrated first on the medication room, supervising as Josef carried the numbered boxes through the lab. Box number three was the first to be removed. Jennifer offered to help.

"There's nothing for you to do," Kane said. "You may as well go home. Clinic as usual tomorrow. Eight-thirty." Somehow, Nurse Kane seemed less rigid, not so uptight, though her voice conveyed little emotion.

Jennifer had wanted to gain access to the Xerox machine inside the clinic suites. She'd hoped to copy the appointment sheets filling one coat pocket, and leave the originals behind for Kane to find. Instead, she nodded politely and left.

At home, Jennifer carefully searched the names in the appointment book. As before, she recognized many of them, but could not find Laniet Teague, number 997. Maybe the alcoholic mother had been wrong. She could have confused their clinic with any of several others: neurology, drug rehabilitation, medicine, ad infinitum. Except for the number. And 997 didn't appear beside any other patient's name. Suddenly Jennifer realized she hadn't noticed Lisa Waters' name, as she had when she scanned the books that day in the clinic. She checked again. Lisa Waters wasn't there. Something heavy sank to the pit of Jennifer's stomach, like a lead ship in a bottomless sea. What had Lisa's number been? She searched her mind frantically. One-oh-two-something. Seven? Nine? Or was it an even number? Six, maybe. Or two. She grabbed a pen and went through the pages again for January, checking off each number in sequence. To her dismay, all the numbers were there, from 1020 through 1030, but the name Lisa Waters didn't exist.

Frustrated, Jennifer threw the pages aside on the sofa and paced her small room, staring out the window as tiny whirling snowflakes bounced off her windowpane.

As the snow began to accumulate outside at dusk, Maria Ortez felt someone gently shake her shoulder. She bolted upright, instantly awake.

"Dr. Traymore is here, Mrs. Ortez."

Maria stood as the tall, thin surgeon entered the waiting room in the children's orthopedic ward. "How he es?" she asked, fearful.

Traymore smiled, deepening the heavy creases in his long face. His voice was incongruously high, like that of a thirteen-year-old boy entering puberty. "The infection's responding," he said. "But he's weak. Lost a lot of blood for a little tyke."

"I give a pint to the blood bank," Maria quickly answered.

Traymore closed his eyes, nodded. "I know. He's getting a transfusion now. Packed cells.

Maria didn't understand.

"Blood," Traymore said. "A special kind, sort of concentrated."

Tears welled up in Maria's eyes again. "His foot?"

"Now, now, don't cry. We're going to save the foot. It's only the one toe he lost."

Maria sank back to the couch, suddenly hot and faint. She shook her head from side to side. "He gonna walk cripple?"

Traymore's high voice hesitated, forced a short laugh meant to reassure. "Of course not. Nobody really needs a big toe. He'll walk just like you and me. Normal."

Maria wiped the tears from her cheek with her sleeve.

"You go home now," Traymore said. "You'll need your rest when he leaves the hospital."

She shook her head violently. "I stay," she declared, her tone leaving little room for argument.

Traymore sighed. "He's a good baby, Maria. Strong. He'll be fine."

Maria nodded, looked up. "He never even cried."

David West called Jennifer just before seven that evening. "Neilson's on the PBS station at seven-thirty. Come on over and watch."

Jennifer arrived at West's Hanover House apartment twenty minutes later, sipped a glass of white wine, and agreed on Chinese food for dinner. David phoned in the order.

Dr. Neilson repeated much of what he had said the evening before. He looked secure and professional on camera, in a gray pinstripe suit and gray tie that matched his sideburns. His laugh lines showed up on the screen more than in person. The interviewer, an intense dapper Englishman in his late forties, commented on the sudden overwhelming interest in a medicine to relieve pain.

"The interest has always been there," Neilson said. "This is the first time a foolproof drug has been found."

The interviewer showed film clips of the crowds around New Hope Hospital, asked Neilson if he thought such a response healthy.

"I think it's a damned shame it's necessary," Neilson said. "Opain should be released for production immediately. Suffering people wouldn't have to resort to mob action. They could get it from their own doctors."

"I understand two people were trampled outside your hospital this morning," the Englishman said. "Badly injured."

Neilson winced visibly. "I hadn't heard. I'm very sorry."

"Doctor, you said earlier that Opain would be available in certain foreign countries within weeks. Have you sold the formula to a pharmaceutical company? Do you have a licensing agreement?"

Neilson sipped a glass of water, set it down. "I am making available a small quantity of Opain to an international drug company only for testing. I will personally license and oversee distribution throughout the world."

"Then nobody has an exclusive arrangement with you?"

"Absolutely not. I want Opain to be available to the people of the world. Perhaps many companies will manufacture and distribute it."

"Isn't it true, Dr. Neilson, that your work has been very generously funded by one specific company?"

Neilson nodded. "True. And they were well aware of my feelings about exclusive licensing agreements and ownership of the formula."

"You sound very altruistic, doctor. But don't you stand to reap rather handsome rewards from your discovery?"

Neilson turned to the host. "Several million dollars, I imagine. If you were in chronic, unbearable pain right now, what would you pay for immediate and absolute relief?"

"Well, I . . . How do you put a price on suffering?"

Neilson nodded. "You don't. At least, I won't. To a suffering oil sheikh a single dose of Opain might be worth millions of dollars. To a bedridden arthritic widow on Social Security, maybe her meager monthly allotment." He shook his head. "I won't have it auctioned to the highest bidder. I will see that it's made available for all who need it, at a price they can afford."

Jennifer was moved by Neilson's passion. He *was* a man obsessed. But she had seen his other side as well, the human part. Somehow, the combination made her proud to know such a man. To share a little bit of his glory. "He's very good," she said.

West agreed, answered the door, and began unpacking steaming white cartons of mouth-watering Chinese food. He set two plates on the coffee table in front of the sofa.

When Neilson's interview ended, Jennifer broached

the subject of her concern as they ate, West sitting yoga-style on the floor opposite her. West reaffirmed that he had never seen Laniet Teague or Lisa Waters in the clinic.

"I believe they were both patients there," Jennifer said. "I know Lisa Waters was. I examined her. She just disappeared."

"They often do," West said, taking another helping of fried rice.

"David, I stole the papers out of the appointment book today. To check."

He grinned. "You're really hung up on this, aren't you?"

"I'm concerned. I think Nurse Kane removed their names from the book."

"Why? Do you think Kane sneaked around and killed them or something? Were they prettier than she is?"

Jennifer poked at her food. "Be serious, David. Maybe something happened to them. Like your brain-tumor patient, Heath."

"So Kane buried their bodies in an eerie haunted graveyard during a howling midnight thunderstorm and erased their names from her appointment book, which nobody ever sees or cares about anyway."

Jennifer pushed her plate away, sat back against the sofa.

"Hey," West said. "I'm kidding. Come on, tell me the rest."

She sat silently for a moment, watching him eat. "There isn't any rest. It's all I've got. But maybe she's trying to hide something. Cover it up. Maybe the drug didn't work on them. Made them sick."

"Then Neilson would know, wouldn't he? Do you believe he'd be a part of a cover-up?"

Jennifer pushed a hangnail back with her thumbnail. "No."

West got up from his cross-legged position on the floor, sat beside her. "Jennie, two girls in the entire city of New York decided not to come back to the clinic. Lost to follow-up, as we say. Maybe they moved, died, got married, ran away, or just forgot to come back. It's no big deal, sweetheart. Okay?"

After a long pause, Jennifer asked, "Have you ever had an affair with Nurse Kane?"

West laughed. "That's ridiculous."

"Have you?"

"Of course not. Surely I could do better than that."

Jennifer silently agreed. But she still couldn't figure him out. "You know she's interested, don't you?"

"Jennie, she's only interested in Neilson, if anybody."

Jennifer sipped at her wine. On an impulse she asked, "David, are you really as naive as you act? Or are you a super con man?"

"What's that supposed to mean?"

"How old are you? Thirty? Thirty-one?"

"Thirty-three," he said.

"You must be aware of how women react to you. The nurses. Probably your women patients. Sometimes you seem so overconfident you're almost arrogant. Other times, you seem totally unaware."

He cleared his throat before answering. "I've been around some."

She sat back and watched his discomfort. "You should have had a sister," she said, smiling. "To teach you about women."

After a moment he said quite seriously, "I guess I've spent too many hours studying. There wasn't much time left over."

Whether it was an act or not, she believed him. "Come here," she whispered.

If he was inexperienced, it didn't show. His lips were hungry and searching, filling her with desire, and his arm tightened around her back just before she started to pull away. Suddenly his hair felt full and thick in her fingers, his lips were on her ears, her neck, and deft hands opened her blouse, his fingers warm and eager on her flesh. She pulled back, her chest heaving, and searched his face. The strong angles, flashing eyes, full, parted lips. His nostrils flared in time with her own breathing, and his teeth appeared one by one in a slow, confident smile. "Who needs a sister?" he asked in a husky voice. "You'll do just fine."

Torn between guilt and desire, Jennifer turned away and stood, buttoning her blouse, suddenly aware of her own wetness. "You learn a little too fast," she managed. "And I must go."

He came up behind her, arms encircling her waist. "I wish you'd stay."

Before she could answer, the doorbell rang. Jennifer quickly tucked in her blouse and turned to look out the window as West answered the door. She heard his invitation for someone to come in, and heard a soft female voice decline, saying she'd come back later. Jennifer looked around in time to recognize the long black hair and shapely legs as the pretty nurse walked away.

Frustrated and confused, Jennifer gathered up her purse and sweater. Despite West's objections, she said she had to leave. At the door, she forced her voice to remain calm, and said, "I've got to see those computer tapes, David. Will you help me?"

At eight-thirty that evening, Nurse Kane stormed into the clinic and down the hall behind the animal lab. "What do you mean, gone?" she demanded as Josef opened the door.

"She got loose," he said. "I untied one arm like always, the one without the cast on it, so she could eat dinner. The other one started to yell, and I went to check on her, worried about her heart."

Kane pushed past him down the narrow hall toward Laniet Teague's room. Josef followed, explaining. "I wasn't gone that long, but when I came back, the room was empty. Straps untied, and her clothes gone."

Kane glowered at him. "You fool. She could be anywhere in the hospital."

"Or the city," he said.

"Did she have a coat?" Kane asked.

"No."

"Then she won't get far in this weather. It's a blizzard outside." Kane slumped against Laniet's empty bed.

"Damn. Why now?" she said to herself. "Another month. Maybe a week, and it wouldn't matter." She turned to Josef. "I'll go through the hospital. You check the streets in the area. The bars. Anyplace she might go to get warm."

Josef nodded, turned to go.

"If we're lucky," Kane said, "she'll jump in front of a truck."

12

---·•◦•◦•·---

Wednesday morning, Jennifer showed her I.D. and passed through the police barricade that cordoned off the corridor to the pain clinic. Nurse Kane stood at her repaired reception counter stiff and starched, ready for business as usual, seemingly unaware of the commotion outside. David West was nowhere around.

With a minimum of words, Jennifer hung up her coat and scarf and went to work. Apparently Kane had limited appointments to patients already established in the clinic. Number 1024, Mary, begrudgingly admitted that her shingles pain was "maybe a little better," though it tested out at only level 1 on the pain machine. Mary discreetly asked in a whisper if she had been on Neilson's wonder drug. Jennifer said she didn't know, though she was almost certain Mary had been receiving injections of sterile water.

"It's a wonderful thing," Mary said as she was leaving. "God bless you doctors."

Kid Foster smiled his boyish smile at Jennifer, stripped off his shiny blue parka, and sat before the pain machine with muscles bulging in his arms and shoulders beneath a tight blue-and-white-striped T-shirt. "Feels real good," he drawled, tilting his blond head from side to side. His tests showed no pain in his neck. At a pain-stimulus level of 24, Kid Foster grinned. "Can't hardly feel it," he said. His blood pressure, pulse, and respiration were perfectly normal. Jennifer asked him to come back in a week.

"I seen that Dr. Neilson on TV," Foster said. "Tell him I'm with him a hunnerd percent." The shiny-slick material of his royal-blue jacket looked as though it would split across his hulking shoulders as he zipped up the front. "When I'm champ, tell him he's got a ringside seat anytime he wants."

Jennifer's next patient was Stephanie Adams, who entered smiling, brushing at the snow-damp scarf she removed from her dark hair. "It's just unreal," Steph said. "Dr. Pearl, even, couldn't believe it. The whole root canal, and I didn't feel a thing. I still didn't like that drill whining in my head like a two-hundred-pound mosquito caught in my ear, but I didn't jump or squirm or anything. I told him it had to be that miracle drug I saw on TV, that Opain. Well, anyway . . ."

Stephanie's pain threshold had gone up six points. Jennifer shook her head in amazement, asked Stephanie to return in a week.

After lunch, Jennifer made a quick trip to check on Melanie Wardner. Alone in her room, Melanie was propped up in bed asleep, an untouched tray of something pureed green and brown on the hospital tray cantilevered over her legs. Melanie opened her small eyes when Jennifer called her name, and tried to speak. Her voice was airy and distant, as though her vocal cords didn't quite have the strength to produce sound. Jennifer tried to feed her with the clean spoon on the tray, got two spoonfuls down before Melanie fell asleep again. Jennifer asked a fat, huffy aide to please try to feed Melanie, and checked her chart at the bustling nurses' station. Melanie's blood count and chemistries were normal. Jennifer made the standard brief note on the chart, indicating only that Melanie appeared to be free of pain. "Comfortable. In no acute distress."

On the fifth floor, Jennifer arrived just as the curly-haired plastic-surgery resident orated ebullient orders to a diminutive Filipino nurse to get Mr. Jennings out of bed and into the hydrotherapy tank across the hall.

"He's doing great," the resident said, beaming proudly. "We've got the best burn unit in the city."

Jennifer tried not to let her own discomfort show when Jennings, a stiff, scab-and-ointment-covered leather man, hobbled to the door, supported by the tiny nurse.

Jennifer forced a smile. "You're moving very well, Mr. Jennings."

Jennings looked at her with his eye, held to the door frame for support. "Feel better," he managed, without moving his masklike face. He limped barefoot across the hall where the nurse led him. The resident followed as Jennings disappeared through the door to the hydrotherapy room.

"Put 'em in the tank, the water swirls off the scabs and bacteria every time," the resident announced. "Try the high setting for ten minutes," he commanded the nurse as he closed the door behind him. "If he can't take it, we'll do medium for fifteen."

Jennifer spun around to leave, but immediately covered her mouth with one hand and gagged. In front of her right shoe was a perfect cast of a man's blood-smeared foot. The burned skin of the entire bottom of Mr. Jennings' left foot had stuck to the tile floor, pulled off. Bloody footprints marked his erratic path from that point to the closed door beyond. Jennifer leaned against the wall for support until her nausea gradually subsided, trying to force the picture from her mind. When she could, she told the nurse at the station what had happened and left, careful to step well over the bottom of Mr. Jennings' foot on the way out. She passed an unconcerned janitor with mop and bucket near the elevator.

In the lab that afternoon, Josef appeared to be behind schedule, and was hurriedly filling the medication reservoirs of the cages when Jennifer entered. He didn't grin, for which she was grateful. She was in no mood for the animal experiments, and kept wondering how much it must hurt to have the sole of your foot peeled off, especially right after it had been so painfully burned. She shuddered again at the thought. Josef interrupted her macabre visions to pour a clear liquid into the reservoir of the cage beside her. Jennifer saw the number 3 taped to the side of the plastic bottle, wondered if it indicated Opain, the same as the medication box she had seen before. Reluctantly she switched on the power console in front of her and turned the dial to 1. The white rat responded as expected: pressed its lever and lapped up its reward. She took it only up to level 6 and flipped off the machine, though the animal sat calmly, as though questioning her unwillingness to play the game. A horrendous crash caused Jennifer to almost jump off her chair, and she wheeled around to see Josef standing rigidly in the center of the room, a spilled metal tray of feeding bowls and instruments clattering around his feet. His long face was contorted and drawn, as if in pain, and his hands shook uncontrollably.

"Josef," she called, quickly going to him. "What's wrong?"

He took a great inhalation and opened his eyes, his face slowly relaxing. "It's nothing," he managed, stooping to retrieve the fallen supplies with shaking hands.

"You're trembling all over," Jennifer said. "And you're perspiring."

Without looking up, he shook his head. "It's okay," he said harshly. He stood and started for the door.

Before Jennifer could react, the door swung open, Nurse Kane almost running into Josef. As he tried to hurry out, Kane grasped his arm, quickly surveying him. "You know better," she said, flushing.

"I've got to try," he said, a husky whisper.

Jennifer took a step toward them, almost tripping over a metal bowl on the floor.

"What are you doing here?" Kane demanded, glaring at Jennifer.

"I'm supposed to be here," Jennifer countered. "And he's ill." She nodded toward Josef, his drenched back to her, his shoulders slumped.

Kane quickly recovered her composure and spoke to

Josef, her tone softer. "You shouldn't try to work when you have the flu. I'll give you an antibiotic." To Jennifer she said, "I'll take care of it. When you finish up here, you can go." And she guided Josef into the hall and shut the door.

On the way out, Jennifer paused at the door to the room that housed Neilson's computer. A quick glance verified that nobody was around. She put her ear to the door, heard nothing inside. As gently as possible she grasped the metal doorknob, turned it slowly to the right. The latch clicked, making her heart race, her mouth dry. Again checking both ends of the corridor, she pressed forward against the door. It didn't budge. She tried harder, leaning her shoulder into the stubborn door. Damn. The upper lock was thrown, probably a deadbolt. She glanced at the circular brass plate, saw the name Siegel. Frustrated at being so close, she tied her scarf around her head and left. She went out a side exit from the hospital to avoid any remaining crowds on First Avenue. While police efforts had done little to dissuade the throngs of anxious people in pain, word had spread that no Opain was available at the hospital. Radio and TV stations repeated that message at hourly intervals throughout the day. Regardless, a few hundred hopeful souls came in the morning seeking help. Many stayed all day, stamping their feet and shuffling about on the frozen sidewalks for warmth.

Outside, fresh white snow blanketed the city, still falling in great floating flakes. Jennifer closed her eyes and listened to the near-silence the snow had brought. Even the usual cacophony of taxi horns seemed muted, soaked up into the peaceful white, like moisture into a thirsty sponge. Jennifer enjoyed the crisp windless chill on her cheeks, and took a great lungful of the cleansed air. She tested the grip of her snowboots on the sidewalk and headed across the avenue for a brisk walk around the block. After a few minutes her thoughts strayed to her evening in David West's apartment. Though initially annoyed that he'd offered no explanation of why the pretty nurse had come to the door—she hadn't asked—she had to admit she held no claims on West. And didn't really want any, she decided. She'd made her commitment to Steve. But she did enjoy West's company. As a friend. And there was nothing wrong with having a friend.

While Jennifer walked and sorted out her thoughts, Laniet Teague awoke in a tousled low bed in Greenwich Village. She swung her legs over the side, glanced at the plaster splint on her toe, stood and stretched, yawning. She stopped to stare at her nude reflection in the wavy mirror on the dresser, amused at the sight of her tangled red hair and casted right arm. She padded through the bedroom door into the light of the small living room beyond. The strange furnishings were meager, chipped and sagging, and the long-haired young man on the settee with a cigarette dangling almost into his beard was sallow and thin. His bony shoulders hunched forward under a stained sweatshirt as he watched a game show in the cold room. He removed the cigarette from his mouth, took a swig from a can of beer, and looked up. Laniet tossed her long red hair off her shoulders and smiled, sucking in her flat stomach and lifting her chest. She turned sideways in the door, crooked her finger at the man, and winked.

"Aww, no," he cawed. "Not again."

"Please? Just once more."

He shook his hairy face. "No way, baby. You almost tore it off."

Laniet nibbled at a corner of her mouth. "I'll be gentle," she said. "If you promise to hurt me this time."

He turned back to the television set, coughed. "Maybe you just ought to go."

She moved in front of the TV and bent forward, rotating her shoulders in slow, easy circles, her full breasts swinging like soft pendulums before his eyes.

"Just 'cause I gave you a ride, let you stay the night, don't mean you live here, you know."

She cooed, licked her lips. "I'll let you whip me again."

He spit on the floor, wiped his mouth on the back of his hand. "I should call in some buddies. Black boots. Whips and chains. You'd like that, huh?"

Laniet pressed her weight forward on her broken toe, shivered a little. "Okay," she said.

Jennifer arrived home at three-fifteen, dusted snow from her scarf and coat, and hung them in the bathroom. She glanced at the New York *Times*, saw Dr. Franklyn Neilson's name and photograph on the first page. The article reported his discovery of Opain and his objection that the FDA would prevent U.S. citizens from obtaining the miracle drug. The head of the FDA was quoted as being critical of Neilson's premature announcement, and reaffirmed that no drug would be released without animal and clinical trials to prove its effectiveness and safety. Neilson was reported to have been inundated with calls and telegrams from people in pain as well as from pharmaceutical companies throughout the world. He declined to state what arrangements had been made for marketing Opain, saying negotiations were under way with several major manufacturers. The administrator of New Hope University Hospital would say only that Dr. Neilson's work was done privately and had no official connection with the hospital except that Neilson headed up the Pain Control Clinic and was on the staff at the hospital and university. He emphasized that Opain was not available at the hospital, and would not be until it received approval from the FDA. The article further stated that demonstrations had occurred outside the FDA offices in Washington, D.C., and isolated protest marches had occurred throughout the country on a smaller scale than in New York City. Neilson was scheduled to appear on *The Tonight Show* this evening.

Jennifer finished the article, flipped through the rest of the paper. On impulse, she looked up the number Mrs. Teague had given her and dialed, asked if Laniet had come home or if she had heard from her.

"Not a word," the woman slurred. "Think she'd have the decency to call her own mother."

Jennifer asked if she had ever stayed away this long.

The woman hesitated. "One time, a week, I think. No, almost two. I just hope she'd not dead somewhere."

"Why do you say that?"

Mrs. Teague coughed into the phone, a wheezing rattle. "She almost died one time. Drugs."

"She took too much?"

"Yeah. That's when they called me."

Jennifer said she was sorry, would check back later.

"That's what I told that other woman that called. Probably on the drugs again. Oh, Lord, I never could do anything with that girl."

"What woman?" Jennifer asked.

"From the hospital."

"Who was it? Do you remember her name?"

"Don't think she ever said. Just called to see if Laniet was here."

Jennifer said good-bye, hung up, and stared at the phone for several minutes. She dialed Maria Ortez's number, let it ring till she was certain nobody was there. At three-fifty that afternoon she left her apartment and took the Second Avenue bus downtown. It didn't make sense that Maria wouldn't be home in such freezing weather. She surely wouldn't take her infant son out in this.

Jennifer stood in the crowded bus amid silent, rosy-cheeked passengers who seemed huddled together for warmth like Alaskan sled dogs, alert, antagonistic, but willing to endure close proximity to avoid freezing in the snow outside. Nobody made eye contact. She exited and walked through dirty slush to Maria's address. Upstairs, there was no answer to her knock. The bartender downstairs had no idea when Maria came or went, said he didn't know her. Jennifer left a note on Maria's door and took the First Avenue bus back uptown, dismayed and concerned. Maybe Maria had gone to stay with a relative, she decided. But she had promised to come by the clinic during the week. At home, Jennifer put Juan's gift-wrapped packages back in her closet and boiled water for a cup of tea. She watered her sagging African violets. At five-thirty she knocked on the building super-intendent's door to ask when the extra lock would be installed on her door.

The thick, balding man held his ever-present beer in one hand, scratched at something in his undershirt with the other. "I been real busy," he said. "Pipes broke in the basement. I'll try to get you tomorrow. Okay?"

Jennifer said it was, but silently resented having to slide her desk against the door every night. Upstairs, she called David West's number. She would offer to buy the pizza if they could watch Neilson on *The Tonight Show*. A female voice answered David's phone.

"He isn't here," the voice said. "Leave a message?"

Jennifer started to say no, pictured the pretty brunette nurse with the long swinging legs. "Dr. Barton," she said. "He knows the number."

Jennifer fixed a tuna salad, ate it with a hard-boiled egg and tea at seven-thirty. West returned her call at eight. "Sorry, Jennie, I've got plans already."

"It's okay," she said. "I should get to bed early anyway." She hung up, depressed, and forced herself to think about how she could possibly get into the computer room at the lab. Neilson, Kane, and probably Josef had keys. Somehow she had to get one for herself. She tried Maria's number once more, finally took a bath and went to bed at ten.

As the prerecorded *Tonight Show* aired in New York, Dr. Franklyn Neilson unbuckled his seat belt in the first-class section of the return flight from Los Angeles. He smiled at the lithe blond stewardess, accepted a glass of champagne.

"You're Dr. Neilson, aren't you?"

"And your name tag says you're Diana."

"Anderson. Diana Anderson." She lowered her eyelashes, raised them again. "It must be a great feeling to invent the perfect pain drug. I saw you on TV."

Neilson's laugh lines deepened. "When you finish serving drinks, come sit down and I'll tell you about it."

At about the time Dr. Neilson got the New York lay-
over number of the fascinated young stewardess somewhere over Iowa, Lisa Waters awoke in a cold sweat in
her bed near the abandoned morgue of New Hope University Hospital. Somehow, the blanket covering her had
slipped down, and her room was freezing. Erratic bursts
of shivers shook her body, and she heard her own teeth
clatter together. Her hands and feet were so tightly
bound she could hardly move. She tried to remember
her fading dream and the delicious raw pain she felt
when she held the button down and forced the numbers
up to 23. She felt the cold gradually go away as she
called back the experience and felt her muscles tense. A
surge of anger warmed her further when she thought of
how Josef had turned off the wonderful machine early
that evening when she had barely started to enjoy it.
And she hadn't even blacked out. Lisa twisted and
strained at the straps on her wrists, heard them creak,
felt her shoulder muscles cramp, begin to ache. It felt
good. But it wasn't enough. She couldn't let him turn the
machine off again. It wasn't fair. She thought about the
way he looked at her each time he put her in the chair.
The way his hand always brushed against her breast or
touched her flank. She could tell what the enormous man
wanted. The way he licked his lips, and from his funny
eyes. Maybe if she offered him what he wanted, he'd not
turn off the machine next time. Maybe she could get up
to 23 for real, like in her dream. She heard her own tiny
voice call out in the darkness, "Josef? Are you there?"
There was no reply. After a while, Lisa swallowed an
enormous lump in her throat and began to cry.

13

In clinic Thursday morning, Jennifer asked Nurse Kane about Josef.

"He's fine," Kane said. "A touch of twenty-four-hour flu."

Just then, Kane answered the phone and handed it to Jennifer. Jennifer didn't recognize the name, Julia Rodriguez.

"I'm the case worker assigned to Maria Ortez," Miss Rodriguez said.

"She's on welfare?"

"She applied for benefits while she was in the hospital. For her son, Juan. I've been by her place several times, but I can't catch her at home. I found a note on her door with your name and number. Can you help me?"

Jennifer said she didn't know where to reach Maria. "Maybe she's staying with a relative."

Papers rattled in the background while Miss Rodriguez paused. "Her application doesn't list any relatives."

Nurse Kane put a chart on the desk beside Jennifer. "Miss Rodriguez," Jennifer said, "I'm worried that something may have happened to Maria. Please call me if you locate her. I'll do the same for you."

At ten-fifteen, Jennifer looked up from where she

stood beside Nurse Kane at the reception counter, to see Ella Lu Mavis being wheeled toward her in a wheelchair. Ella Lu was perspiring heavily, looked even skinnier than Jennifer remembered. A bearded Puerto Rican orderly asked, "You Dr. Barton?"

When Jennifer said she was, he turned and left. Jennifer asked Ella Lu what was wrong.

"Don't feel good," she said. "My stomach."

Jennifer felt the girl's forehead. "You're burning up. Let's get you inside."

In the examining room, Ella Lu told Jennifer what she felt. "Just hot, then freezing to death. Makes me shake all over. Can't hardly stand up."

"Does anything hurt?" Jennifer asked.

Her big round suspicious eyes looked up at Jennifer. "No."

Ella Lu's temperature was one hundred and four degrees. Though she denied pain, her abdominal muscles were rigid, boardlike. Her pulse and respiration were fast, in keeping with her fever.

"Went to the emergency room," Ella Lu said. "Told 'em to call you. Ain't lettin' nobody cut on me."

"Did they suggest surgery?"

"They would. That one doctor wanted to cut out my tubes that time."

While Jennifer examined Ella Lu, Nurse Kane took a call outside from the emergency-room nurse. "We sent a patient up there, Ella Lu Mavis. Dr. Rayle just checked her X rays and lab, says she's got a ruptured appendix. He wants to know if she'd had anything that might keep her from showing any pain?"

"She's had nothing from here," Kane said. "What does she look like?"

"You mean you haven't seen her? A skinny black kid. Kind of a big head, big brown eyes."

"She was here earlier," Kane said. "She left."

"Well, she won't get far," the nurse said. "She's got a raging peritonitis. Infection all over her abdomen. If she comes back, call us. She's got to have emergency surgery."

Kane said she would, hung up. She dialed Josef's number in the lab, spoke briefly with him.

Meanwhile, Ella Lu told Jennifer her other problems. "And Mama threw me out. She's religious."

"Why?" Jennifer asked.

"Yesterday." She shook her outsized head, shrugged. "Found out I was doin' it for money." Her eyes quickly checked Jennifer's reaction.

Jennifer took the girl's hot hand, helped her sit up on the examining table. "Ella Lu, you've got a serious infection. Maybe it's PID, maybe not. It could be your appendix. You're sure it didn't hurt when I touched your stomach?"

She blinked. "I'm sure."

"I'll call the emergency room or the gynecology clinic. You've got to let them treat you."

Ella Lu stared at the floor, looked up again, sweat streaming down her forehead and face. "Don't let 'em cut me."

Nurse Kane opened the door and interrupted their conversation. "The emergency room called, wants to do some more tests. I'll take her down."

"It's all right," Jennifer assured Ella Lu. "I'll check on you. They probably just want to give you some antibiotics."

Ella Lu reluctantly got into the wheelchair, allowed Nurse Kane to wheel her out the door. Kane turned before she left. "Your next patient is in room two," she told Jennifer.

When Jennifer finished seeing the remainder of her appointments, she called the emergency room, asked about Ella Lu.

"She walked out, I guess," the nurse said.

Jennifer asked her to explain.

"Nurse Kane left her parked in the waiting room. It's a madhouse down here. Patients everywhere. When I went to call her, she was gone. I thought maybe she was back up there, or in X Ray."

Jennifer was dumbfounded. She hurried to the reception desk, asked Nurse Kane about Ella Lu.

"I took her to the emergency room. That's all I know. *They* lost her."

Jennifer felt a rush of heat in her face. "That poor girl has a serious infection. Maybe peritonitis. She could die."

Kane blinked once, narrowed her eyes. "I know that. I spoke with the emergency room. She has a ruptured appendix. The girl walked out. She's deathly afraid of surgery."

Exasperated, Jennifer raced to the overflowing emergency room. She finally cornered a frenetic nurse long enough to piece together what had happened. Apparently Nurse Kane brought Ella Lu to the emergency room as requested. Kane had been told that the girl had a ruptured appendix. But only an empty wheelchair was found when they went for Ella Lu. None of the other waiting patients remembered seeing the girl.

After lunch, Jennifer called Ella Lu's mother.

"She ain't here, won't be here," Mrs. Mavis intoned.

"Ella Lu is very ill, Mrs. Mavis. She desperately needs an emergency operation."

"Call her pimp, then. Tell him." Mrs. Mavis hung up.

Jennifer searched the hospital corridors and the streets outside, but found no trace of Ella Lu Mavis. She could only hope that the frightened girl would come back, or go to another hospital in time.

In the lab, Josef told Jennifer there were no experiments for the day. He looked perfectly all right.

"How are you feeling?" Jennifer asked.

"Fine," he said, busying himself sweeping the floor.

Jennifer started to ask about his bout with the flu, but sensed his reluctance to talk. She started for the door. Just as she reached for the handle, Josef called her name.

"Yes?" she asked, turning.

He smiled a genuine smile. "Thank you for caring," he said.

She was taken by surprise at his sudden warmth. "You're welcome," she said, and left.

Since no experiments were set up for the afternoon, Jennifer made early rounds. Mr. Jennings seemed stiffly comfortable, and had received a skin graft to his left foot along with excision and grafting of obvious third-degree burns on his legs and arms. Jennifer noticed large chunks of flesh missing from his chest, and one dusky-blue skin graft neatly stitched like football lacing on his forehead. He appeared much thinner than she remembered.

On the fourteenth floor, a pale, drained Melanie Wardner was raised up in her electric bed and spoke briefly with Jennifer. "I'm so tired," Melanie rasped in a faint voice. "It's startin' to hurt a little."

"Is it bad?" Jennifer asked.

Melanie shook her head, pointed to her lower abdomen in the region of her bladder. "Just here."

Jennifer promised to give her something if the pain got worse. "But it's better if you don't take too much."

Melanie nodded, sighed weakly, closed her eyes. "All this for a little pinched pee tube."

"I know," Jennifer said. "If it gets worse, have them call me."

As Jennifer walked out into the corridor, a tall well-dressed girl with a long narrow face, prominent nose, and large round plastic-framed glasses stopped her. "I'm Bea Prentiss," the girl said. "Melanie's roommate. Could I please speak with you?"

After answering Bea's questions about Melanie's surgery and complications, Jennifer invited her for a cup of coffee in the hospital cafeteria.

"She looks so pale," Bea said. "Almost like a different person. Melanie's always been the most alive girl I've ever known. The life of the party. Now she just lies there moaning, or sleeps."

"She's very weak, Bea. Exhausted. It's been rough on her."

Bea stared into her coffee. "Poor kid. She doesn't need this right now."

Jennifer asked her to explain.

Bea hesitated, then spoke. "She was engaged to a fellow from Boston. He broke it off last month and took off with somebody else for Africa, with no warning. A photographic safari."

"I'm sorry."

Bea shrugged. "I would've been devastated. But Melanie took it pretty well. She's always up, you know? Chipper. Always sees the good in things. Constantly doing things for other people, like never forgetting my birthday or my parents' anniversary." Bea removed her enormous glasses and wiped a tear from her cheek. "She'd never admit it, but she's really worried about how she'll ever pay her hospital bill. God, it must be enormous by now. She doesn't have any insurance."

"She could transfer to a cheaper room, or the ward."

Bea shook her head. "Not Melanie. She goes first class, and pays her own way. But she only had a couple of thousand dollars saved up. She must owe fifteen or twenty thousand by now."

Jennifer sighed. "It is very expensive." She sipped her tea, set it down. "She's not having any pain now, Bea. She's over the rough part. And she'll be getting out soon."

Bea took a deep breath, glanced up at Jennifer. "Oh, God, I hope so. She looks so helpless just lying there. Like a little broken bird that fell out of its nest. I used to call her the girl who never sleeps. Work all day, disco all night, come in smiling and happy just in time to change clothes for work again."

Jennifer toyed with her cup. "Has she always had a low tolerance for pain? Cramps, maybe? A toothache?"

Bea shrugged. "She's never been sick. Always said she didn't have time. She exercises, takes vitamins. I don't think she ever considered having pain."

After a moment's silence, Jennifer asked about Melanie's family.

"She hasn't had anybody since she was a kid. Father

disappeared somewhere, mother drank herself to death. Melanie always said she was her own family. Said she pulled herself up by her panty hose. Made it on her own."

"What does she do?"

Bea almost smiled. "One of the most promising commercial artists in the city. She'll be tops someday." Her face slowly twisted and reddened. "If she gets out of here."

Jennifer squeezed the girl's hand. "She will, Bea."

Jennifer left for home early that afternoon. Although the snow had stopped the night before, the skies were thick with clouds from an expected new storm. The sidewalks were wet and slippery, and cold black water spewed from the tires of passing cars. Great puddles made it risky to stand near the corners on First Avenue. In her apartment, Jennifer tried to reach Maria Ortez and Ella Lu. Maria's number didn't answer. Mrs. Mavis slammed the receiver down in Jennifer's ear when she heard her voice. Jennifer fixed a cup of tea and flipped through Thursday's *Times*. The article on Dr. Neilson had moved to an inside page, pretty much repeated what had been said before. Jennifer's eyes stopped on a picture of Kid Foster in the sports section. But her heart sank when she read the caption beneath: "KID FOSTER PARALYZED."

Jennifer bit her lip, felt as if the sofa had suddenly dropped out from under her as she read the details. The twenty-two-year-old fighter who was expected to be a contender for the heavyweight boxing title had suffered a spinal-cord injury during a workout. X rays confirmed a fracture of a vertebra in his neck. He was totally paralyzed from the neck down. His sparring partner was unavailable for comment. Foster had undergone emergency surgery, but his doctors said it was much too early to know whether he might ever regain any use of his arms and legs. They did say he would never fight again. Jennifer dropped the paper on her lap and cried.

She tried to call Dr. Neilson's home number several

times, but it was persistently busy. She finally reached David West a few minutes after five. He agreed to come straight over.

When he arrived, West removed his tie and white jacket, opened the collar of his shirt before taking the seat opposite her. He leaned forward, his face lined with concern. "Jennie, it's not your fault."

"He was my patient."

"But you didn't give him the injection. Besides, it would have happened anyway. He must have had a weak spot, or a ruptured disk."

Jennifer wiped a tear from her cheek with the back of her hand. "If he'd felt the pain, it might have warned him."

West drew a long breath, shook his head.

"There's another one," Jennifer said. "A young black girl who got Opain. She came in with peritonitis today. A ruptured appendix. And she never felt the first pain."

"Then how did you diagnose it?"

"I wasn't sure. She's a prostitute. Has a history of gonorrhea, PID. Emergency-room X rays showed gas in her abdomen."

"Well, at least you found out. Was it ruptured when they got in?"

"They never got to operate. She left. Walked out."

"With a ruptured appendix? You sure?"

Jennifer tucked her feet under her, leaned back on the sofa, sniffed. "David, if it had hurt like they usually do, she would have begged for surgery. Maybe come in before it ruptured. Don't you see?"

West frowned and stood up, walked around the room silently, then asked for a glass of wine.

"In the refrigerator," Jennifer said.

He helped himself, offered to pour her one. "Have you told Neilson?"

"I can't get him," she said. "He's either deluged with calls or has his phone off the hook."

West was silent for a long moment, then asked, "Are you sure they were both on Opain?"

"What else could it be?"

West nodded, sat back. "Probably. But Neilson would know for sure. Or Kane."

"Ha," Jennifer said. "She wouldn't give me the time of day. Maybe you should ask."

"Why me?"

"Oh, David. I never get anything but an icy glare."

"Maybe she's jealous. Thinks you're after Neilson."

Jennifer stopped to think, remembered Kane's voice softening perceptibly when Neilson was present.

West interrupted her thoughts. "Why haven't you put a new lock on your door?"

"The super promised to have it on last Monday. He says he'll do it either tonight or tomorrow morning."

"Make him do it, Jennie. Or I will. Addicts think all doctors and nurses keep drugs in their apartments."

Jennifer half-listened to his warning. She was thinking of something else. "It never occurred to me that not having pain could be bad."

West sipped his wine, studied her face.

"What if nobody ever experienced pain, David? How would you know when you had an infection? An abscessed tooth? Appendicitis?"

"Some kids are born without pain receptors, usually in limited areas of the body, like the hands. They keep injuring themselves. Touching hot stoves, that sort of thing. But they learn."

Jennifer sat forward. "David, I'm worried about Opain. Maybe it's too good."

"Don't be silly. It eventually wears off. Look at the lab animals."

She considered what he'd said. Admitted it was true. "But it didn't wear off fast enough for Kid Foster. Maybe not for Ella Lu."

"Those are two isolated incidents in over a thousand cases, Jennie. It doesn't make it all bad."

She watched his intense face, felt her eyes sting. "Tell that to Kid Foster."

Jennifer refused West's offer to go with her, changed from her whites into her beige skirt and sweater, and took the bus crosstown a little after seven. When she arrived at Roosevelt Hospital, she was directed to Kid Foster's room. When she opened his door, the sight she saw broke her heart. The strapping youth with the slow, easy grin and bulging muscles lay facedown on a tubular steel-and-canvas Stryker frame, perfectly still beneath the sheets, staring at the floor. Jennifer tried to stand where he could see her, since only his eyes seemed to move. A slim girl with long black hair and puffy eyes moved her chair slightly when Jennifer introduced herself, made room.

"Hi," Jennifer finally said.

Kid Foster's blue eyes strained to see her. She couldn't see if he grinned, but his voice didn't. "Hi."

"I just heard," Jennifer said softly. "I'm sorry."

He took a long breath, exhaled. "Thanks."

Jennifer didn't know what to say. The silence in the room was tense, oppressive. She turned to the fragile girl beside her. "He told me about you."

The girl swallowed, dabbed at her eyes with a tissue. "We were supposed to get married next week." Her face crumpled, squeezing large tears onto her salt-tracked cheeks.

"Come on, honey. Don't do that," Foster said.

Jennifer cleared her throat, fought back her own tears. "You're strong, Kid. In good shape. You'll heal fast."

His eyes darted toward Jennifer, back toward the floor he faced. "How do you heal a metal rod in your neck?"

Jennifer felt his depression. His anger. The hopelessness. But she had to ask. "Did you feel anything when it happened?"

This time his eyes didn't move. "I can't feel nothing, lady. Nothing at all."

Jennifer tried to call Dr. Neilson again from the hospital lobby. His line was still busy. She had to tell him about Kid Foster. Ella Lu. She took a taxi to Neilson's apartment building, went upstairs. Neilson answered on her third knock. He seemed genuinely pleased to see her, invited her inside.

Jennifer entered the smoke-stuffy room as Neilson closed the door behind her. There were three other men present, Orientals. One was very much overweight, in a gray business suit and tie, one old and thin with unblinking lizard eyes. Both smoked strong cigarettes; the thin one used a long black cigarette holder. A third man stood to one side of Neilson's velvety room, was short, trim, and so bald his head shone like a brass ball in the light above him. He sported an incongruous Vandyke beard. He bowed politely as Jennifer was introduced. The other two men nodded from where they sat.

"My associate, Dr. Barton," Neilson said.

The fat Chinese man spoke with only a slight accent. "Shall we come back?"

Neilson took Jennifer's London Fog, showed her to a seat. "I'd like her to hear, gentlemen."

The thin old man nodded perceptibly with no change of expression, and the fat man spoke. "We are interested in an exclusive arrangement in our country," he said to Jennifer. He turned to Neilson. "And other countries. Our company is very large. The cost is not important. We prefer to be the only company to have Opain." He turned to the old man, spoke rapidly in Chinese. The old man nodded stiffly, his thin neck hardly touching the edges of his starched white shirt collar.

Neilson sat in a chair beside Jennifer, facing the two men across the glass-topped coffee table. "Gentlemen, your offer is very generous. Before making a final decision, I would like to see your plants, as you suggested. A sufficient quantity of Opain is available for you to confirm my test results. I see no reason why we can't reach a mutually satisfactory agreement."

The fat man again interpreted for the old one, who uttered one terse burst of Chinese. The fat man asked Neilson, "When can we begin our tests?"

Neilson stood. "When your funds arrive at my bank in Switzerland."

After a brief exchange, the Chinese men stood, the fat

one shook Neilson's hand. The other bowed, to Neilson and to Jennifer. "Tomorrow," the fat man said. They were joined by the bald, bearded Chinese man as they left the apartment.

"What's that all about?" Jennifer asked when they were alone.

"Another group after the rights to Opain. They're from Peking."

Jennifer straightened in her chair. "You trust them?"

Neilson laughed. "The old man owns the largest conglomerate in his country, plus holdings throughout the world. They are about to deposit twenty million dollars in gold to my account in Zurich as a show of good faith."

Jennifer whistled. "Before they've even tested Opain?"

Neilson nodded, poured two glasses of champagne. "I showed them the results of my study."

"That doesn't seem very shrewd on their part."

Neilson lifted his glass. "My dear, if Opain didn't work, they would make me beg to give them their twenty million back. Money that big can buy the best professionals."

"You mean they'd kill you?"

Neilson smiled. "Worse. Much worse." He touched his glass to hers. "To Opain," he said.

Jennifer tasted the champagne, felt the bubbles tingle her nostrils. She watched Neilson stare deep into her own eyes, his gaze confident, assured, but warm. She set her glass on the coffee table. "I came here to tell you about two very serious problems," she began. "Opain may be responsible."

Neilson sat silently beside her while she told him about Kid Foster and Ella Lu Mavis. He questioned her about the original pain thresholds of the two patients, his expression one of intense concentration, his brow knotted. "Did they get injections or oral doses?"

Jennifer tried to remember. "Injections, I think. Why?"

Neilson didn't answer right away. He leaned back against the sofa. "I'm not sure. The oral preparation is newer. It's harder to control the dose than with injections." He sat in silence for several moments, turned to Jennifer. "I can't really conclude that Opain caused these problems. A malformed vertebra on the fighter, most likely. A girl with recurrent pelvic infections develops appendicitis." He shook his head. "No. Opain isn't responsible."

Jennifer sensed his internal struggle, detected it in his eyes, his voice. Perhaps it was the only conclusion he could reach. She cleared her throat. "Maybe some pain is good. Necessary."

Neilson's eyes blazed for an instant. "I refuse to accept that."

"But pain is the body's signal that something's wrong. A warning device."

"There are other signals. Fever, swelling, redness, diminished function. Stiffness. People shouldn't have to suffer to know when they're ill."

Jennifer hesitated to push further. She saw the magnitude of his commitment in the intensity of his reaction. "When did you become obsessed with eliminating pain?" she asked softly.

Neilson blinked twice, sipped his champagne, and answered, "Almost since I can remember."

She watched something cloud his eyes for a moment. "Can it be shared, or am I being too personal?"

He stood, poured more champagne, and stared down at her with the half-empty bottle in one hand. "Obsessions don't arrive full-blown," he said. "They grow, like everything else." He returned to his seat beside her.

"How old were you?"

He almost shrugged with his eyes, stared into the fire. "Eighteen. My first year in college."

Jennifer said as little as possible, but encouraged him when he faltered, genuinely interested. She learned of his average Midwestern home, his father's financial setbacks and untimely death. Neilson's voice expressed a certain reverence when he spoke of his mother. His shining light, he said, who encouraged him to study, expected him to be something. Believed he would make her proud.

It was during his first year of college as an engineering student that she became bedridden with rheumatoid arthritis.

"She was forced to quit work, naturally. What little I made waiting tables at school was barely enough for tuition. I had to drop out, go to work to pay the rent and groceries. She deteriorated very rapidly."

"Was she in severe pain?" Jennifer asked.

Neilson's color faded visibly. "Constant."

"I'm sorry."

He shook his head, and his voice had a ragged edge when he spoke. "I didn't mind the work, taking care of her. I got a construction job during the day and hired a woman to stay with her. It was the nights. Listening to her groan and cry. She tried to muffle her sobs, but I'd hear her cry out to her Lord and beg him to take her. To please stop her misery."

"They had pain drugs then," Jennifer said, more a question than a statement.

"Sure. But doctors were afraid of having a patient become addicted. It was a small town. They could lose their licenses."

Neilson's voice was less shaky now. "She was addicted for a while. To morphine. Then they cut her off." He winced visibly, drained his glass. "That was almost worse than the arthritis."

Jennifer touched his hand, fighting to hold back her tears. "How long?"

He grasped her hand and squeezed gently. "It took two years of suffering and withering for her to die. Without a minute's relief. She fell out of bed, fractured her hip, was dead a month later. It was almost a blessing."

"And you?"

He took a deep breath, purged his lungs. "Went back to college to study for medicine. Later, neurophysiology. I started out to be an arthritis specialist. A rheumatologist. But I saw people suffering from hundreds of other illnesses as well. The one thing they all had in common was pain. You know the rest."

Jennifer leaned her head against the velvety backrest. "She'd be very proud of you." A log fell in the fireplace, sputtered, sending a brief but intense shower of yellow and orange sparks up the chimney.

Neilson's pupils widened as he searched the depths of Jennifer's eyes. "A thousand patients have already had relief from their suffering because of Opain."

Jennifer closed her eyes, almost whispered, "And two may have been hurt because of it." She raised her head, met his gaze.

He didn't blink, but his eyes narrowed. "Jennifer, in a war, many suffer. Some die. So that others may live in peace."

"And your war is with pain."

He slowly nodded. "My own mother was the first casualty."

A short time later, Jennifer asked Neilson to drive her home. On the way she asked, "Could I see the results of your study? The computer information?"

Neilson turned the corner onto First Avenue. "Not yet, Jennie. Someday, I'll show you."

"Don't you trust me?"

He patted her knee. "Of course I do. But I had a rather bad experience once because I was naive. It won't happen again."

Alone in her apartment, Jennifer grumbled aloud about the inefficient superintendent's failure to get her lock installed, scooted her desk in front of her door, bathed, and went to bed.

While Jennifer slept, Ella Lu Mavis stared up at harsh fluorescent lights in her sweat-drenched bed near the hospital morgue, bony ankles and wrists bound to the four corners of the bed. Her skin felt on fire, but great shaking chills racked her emaciated body as if the twigs of her skeleton were encased in winter ice. Intravenous fluids dripped rapidly into the veins of both arms, spiked liberally with an antibiotic. Something gurgled near the lower right side of her abdomen, and clumps of blood-tinged green pus advanced slowly into the clear plastic suction tube which extended over the side of the bed from deep inside her abdomen. Her frail ribs seemed to bend with each harsh thrust as her heart pounded unmercifully against her chest. Her great round eyes, black marbles rimmed with white, stared unblinking at the ceiling, wide and wary.

14

Jennifer checked her African violets and left a note on the building superintendent's door in Brigton House early Friday morning when there was no answer to her knock. She was furious at being put off about the lock on her door, tired of sitting backward in her tub each night watching the front door, half-expecting somebody to come crashing through the puny barricade she erected. She took the tired old elevator to the subbasement level and raced through the maze of tunnels to New Hope University Hospital.

Between patients, she used the clinic phone to call Maria Ortez's and Ella Lu Mavis' number. Neither answered. She gave it little thought that her suspension was over, and she was back on the hospital payroll. She used the clinic Xerox machine to make copies of an article she'd found on reconstruction of the vocal cords after cancer surgery, and watched Nurse Kane go in and out of the computer room several times, always locking the door behind her. Jennifer was delighted when the business executive with the lower back pain walked into her exam room smiling and said he had returned to work, felt fine. She had expected no less. The crowds outside had dwindled to a few hangers-on, but most seemed satisfied to wait for appointments to be seen in the pain clinic. Jennifer's thoughts were on the computer and obtaining a copy of the printout of the patients in Neilson's study. Especially Laniet Teague and Lisa Waters. Kane gave her no opportunity.

After a quick lunch, Jennifer checked on Melanie Wardner, concerned that the girl was not regaining her strength, not eating properly. Melanie appeared small and frail in her bed, her color contrasting very little with the stark whiteness of the bed's linens. Jennifer couldn't help remembering the day in the recovery room when six nurses could hardly hold the girl down. Melanie whined faintly in her sleep like a feverish child having a bad dream as Jennifer approached her bed. She jumped, startled, when Jennifer felt for her pulse.

"I didn't mean to scare you," Jennifer said.

One side of Melanie's mouth twitched, almost smiled. "I'm glad it's you," she said.

"How're you feeling?"

Melanie tried to moisten her lips with a gray tongue. "Okay."

Deep vertical lines in Melanie's forehead made Jennifer doubt her answer. "You sure?"

Melanie closed her eyes for a moment. "It hurts pretty bad," she said.

Jennifer saw the resignation in her eyes, almost the way Walter Jackson had looked at her. "Do you need something for the pain?"

"No," the girl whispered. "I can't."

Jennifer listened to drops of urine steadily plopping into the bottle beneath the bed. "What can't you do, Melanie?"

She turned her head on the pillow to look at Jennifer. "I couldn't stand any more."

Jennifer asked her to explain.

"The pain," Melanie said. "I almost craved it. Wanted more." She closed her sunken eyes, rimmed with dark circles, seemed exhausted.

Jennifer wanted to ask other questions, but heard Melanie's breathing change slightly, knew she needed her rest. She tiptoed from the room.

In the burn unit, Mr. Jennings seemed stronger and less stiff than earlier. He said he was comfortable.

"Have you had any feelings that you craved the pain?" Jennifer asked.

Jennings turned his eye toward Jennifer. "If you've ever been burned," he managed very slowly, "you never want to feel anything again. I'd rather die any day than go through that hell."

Jennifer nodded, looked at his greased cracked-leather hide and face, and said good-bye. The most depressing thing, she thought, was that Mr. Jennings would never be normal again. A successful, apparently wealthy and powerful real-estate developer, virtually reduced to a pile of charcoal and smoldering meat. She shuddered to think of the hundreds of reconstructive operations he might have in future years, futile attempts to hide his distorted, scarred features. She wondered what he had looked like before.

In the afternoon lab, Jennifer balked at the experiment set up for her to perform. Actually, the chimpanzee was to perform his own experiment, with Jennifer there to record the results. Though she objected, Josef filled the liquid dispenser.

"Nurse Kane said do it," Josef grumbled.

Jennifer felt her spine stiffen. "And we always do what Nurse Kane orders, don't we?"

His jaw muscles worked as he clenched his teeth for an instant. "Yes, doctor," he said, and left the room.

Reluctantly Jennifer watched the large chimp, about the size of a human dwarf, press the red lever after drinking from the dispenser. He jumped into the air, twirled, and pressed the lever again. Jennifer wrote down the pain-stimulus intensity of level 4 and waited. Minutes later, the chimp waddled to the lever and stimulated himself again, raising the pain intensity to level 5, about as strong as a typical low-back sprain. The chimp held to the sides of the cage and bounced up and down, chattering at Jennifer, almost grinning.

Jennifer brooded and recorded the impatient chimp's

rapid increases of his pain stimulus to level 12, equivalent to a severe attack of migraine headache. The chimp acted almost gleeful, racing back to the lever for more. Jennifer called to Josef to disconnect the power, but he had gone into the back room. The chimp pushed himself up to 18 and chattered noisily, tugging on the sides of the wire cage as if in play. His blood pressure and pulse climbed steadily, rapidly approaching the danger level. Jennifer couldn't bear to let him go higher. His pain was equal to a red-hot tooth abscess, and he seemed to want more. Melanie Wardner's statement flashed across Jennifer's mind: "I craved it. Wanted more."

Jennifer quickly stood and raced out to the desk in the waiting area. Nurse Kane wasn't there. She ran back into the lab, saw that the chimp was leaning against the pain lever, forcing it down, and the digital readout was up to 24. His blood pressure was high enough to blow out a vessel in his brain any minute. She ran to the back of the lab and pounded on the locked door, shouting for Josef. He didn't respond. Frantic, she raced to the cage and searched for a cord to the power supply. Damn. Josef had wired it direct somehow, and though the console was turned off, the crazed chimp was shooting pain to his body as severe as passing a kidney stone. Jennifer's heart pounded in her ears as she searched desperately for a way to stop the chimp's suicidal pain, but she could find no source of the power, no wires leading to or from the cage. The chimp suddenly shrieked and fell to the floor of the cage gasping, and began to twitch. An arm, then one leg, stiff and jerking—like a dog chasing something in its sleep. Jennifer screamed out for Josef again but heard no reply as she helplessly watched the chimp progress to a full-blown epileptic seizure. In desperation she tore open the door to the cage as the chimp dragged his convulsive body toward the pain lever for more, certain to kill himself. She grabbed one hairy arm, felt a hand almost human encircle hers, and pulled the struggling animal from the cage. One spastic long arm wrapped tightly around her leg. The chimp suddenly bared his teeth in an aggressive snarl and began to grunt deep threatening jungle sounds. She fought to hold her white skirt down as the chimp tried to climb her leg, his fury growing. Her desperate efforts to retreat and shake free only pulled him along with her, clinging frantically to her leg, panting like a mad dog in heat. She almost screamed when she tripped over something behind her, felt herself topple backward, flailing her arms wildly to grab a support as the ape shinnied up her leg and under her skirt. A loud crash followed as her hip thudded painfully against a lab table, sprawling her onto the floor. Two white rats raced over her chest and across the floor from their overturned cages, and the crazed chimp lowered his gnashing teeth toward her face, his eyes wild and frenzied, his hot breath rotten, like decaying cabbage.

"I got him," Josef yelled, tugging at the hairy ape from behind.

Jennifer heard a button rip off her white jacket as the chimp clutched at her. Josef fell backward to the floor, grasping the maddened, shrieking chimp firmly around the waist. Josef was up instantly, one hand firmly controlling the animal's head with a thumb in one ear, a finger in the other.

"You all right?" he asked.

Jennifer nodded uncertainly and sat up, taking stock. Frightened and weak, she saw no serious damage. As she stood and brushed off her skirt, her eyes froze on something shiny beneath the console where Josef had fallen. His key ring. The one he wore on his belt. A quick glance told her Josef was in the back room with his hands full. Still trembling from her nightmarish attack, Jennifer grabbed the keys from the floor and raced outside into the hall.

As she approached the computer-room door, Jennifer heard Nurse Kane's voice near the desk. She shoved the keys into her jacket pocket, looked up.

"Two patients for workup," Kane said. "In about twenty minutes."

Jennifer froze, but forced herself to smile, and walked on rubbery legs toward the exam rooms. She couldn't risk being discovered. And Josef was sure to notice he'd lost his keys. He always locked the rear lab door. Jennifer desperately searched her mind. How could she possibly keep his keys? And she didn't even know which of the many keys opened the door to the computer room. She had to do something. Now. So little time.

Searching the room frantically, Jennifer saw the Xerox machine. She glanced toward where Kane stood at the desk, her back toward Jennifer. With trembling fingers, Jennifer lifted the cover of the Xerox machine, spread the keys flat against the plate one at a time, careful to copy both sides of each key, and jammed them back in her pocket. She extracted the copy sheets, folded them hurriedly, and walked back toward the lab. "Forgot my pen," she told Kane.

Josef came from the back room just as Jennifer entered the experimental lab. When he bent to pick up the overturned cage, she set the keys on the floor and shoved them beneath the console with her foot. "Thank you, Josef."

He nodded.

"I suppose he went cage-crazy too," she said sarcastically.

Josef straightened, narrowed his eyes. "I guess so."

Jennifer turned to leave, stopped abruptly. "Aren't those your keys?" she asked, pointing.

Josef mumbled something and stopped to retrieve them, hanging the clip back over his belt as he walked away.

Jennifer cleaned herself up in the bathroom and saw her two consults. The first was a frail woman of twenty-nine who arrived in a wheelchair, her husband anxious and hopeful behind her. Diagnosis, breast cancer with widespread metastases. Her worst pain seemed to come from the cancer eating away at her spine. Jennifer kept her examination and testing as brief as possible, anxious to provide some relief for the woman's intractable pain. "I'm sure we can help you feel better," Jennifer said.

The gaunt young woman raised her head to look at

Jennifer from her wheelchair. Without speaking, she removed her scarf and wig. Beneath, her head was almost bald, only tiny patches of stubby hair remaining on her sallow scalp, a side effect of high doses of chemotherapy. "I have two babies," she said in a thin voice. "I'll try anything."

Jennifer left the room, intending to insist that Nurse Kane give the young mother Opain. There was no need to test the other drugs further. Halfway up the hall, she met Dr. Neilson, smiling and happy.

"You wouldn't believe it, Jennie. They're calling from all over the world. Drug companies, oil sheikhs, ambassadors. Even the FDA wants to see me."

She said that was great, then told him about the poor woman in her examining room. "She's terminal. In unbelievable pain. Can't you treat her outside the study?"

Neilson agreed, removed a glass vial of Opain from his pocket, and handed it to Jennifer. "Give her this," he said. "Tell her to come back only if the pain returns."

Jennifer accepted the vial and thanked him. The picture of the crazed chimpanzee flashed before her eyes as she started to turn. "Are you sure it's safe?" she asked.

Neilson smiled, patted her arm. "Do you have anything better?" He closed his eyes and nodded. "Give it to her. Let her enjoy her babies before she dies."

Jennifer agreed, then added, "I need to talk with you when you have time. I'm concerned about—"

Neilson cut her off, touching her cheek. "Later," he said. "Use your best judgment on the patients. I've got a million things to do." And he was gone, white coat flowing behind his elegant form.

After giving the injection, Jennifer saw her second patient, a husky cabdriver with persistent neck pain following a whiplash injury. Jennifer listened patiently to the entire story of how some idiot truck driver rammed into his cab from the rear.

"And he didn't have insurance. Can you believe that? I'm out of work three months, and he didn't even have insurance."

The man tested out at pain level 8 on the machine.

Nurse Kane went into the back room for his medication, and Jennifer left.

It was just after four that afternoon when Jennifer got the last of the keys made from her Xerox copies. She'd had each of the others made at different locations, rather than try to explain why she needed so many. This locksmith's expression was as questioning as the others when he saw the imprint on the paper.

"My roommate made a Xerox copy of her key for me," Jennifer said nonchalantly. "It's the only one we have since I lost mine, but the man in the restaurant next door said if anybody could do it, you could."

By four-twenty, Jennifer had exact duplicates of Josef's set of keys. She returned to her apartment building and went down to the dank tunnel toward the clinic. As she hoped, the clinic was locked and deserted.

To be certain nobody was around, Jennifer knocked on each of the doors to the clinic and lab. She would say she had forgotten her scarf if anybody answered. Nobody did. Her mouth felt as dry as if it were packed with dental cotton when she approached the door to the computer room. She held her breath and glanced up and down the hall before taking the keys from her bag. Her hand was freezing and shaky as she inserted the keys into the upper lock one at a time. Three of them were for Siegel locks, she had been told. The second key fit. Just as she began to turn the key, the sound of heels striking the hallway floor echoed from near the elevators. Jennifer pulled out the key and flattened herself against the wall instantly, listening, her heart racing. Somebody laughed in the distance, and two sets of footsteps disappeared in the opposite direction.

Moments later, Jennifer slipped into the computer room and eased the door shut behind her. She groped for the light switch and turned it on. The computer was smaller than she had imagined, about the size of a small refrigerator, with a keyboard like a typewriter. Now all she had to do was figure out how to work it. She shuffled through papers stacked on the desk beside the computer, hoping to find instructions, anything that might give her a clue. She froze when a door slammed somewhere down the hall, and she immediately flipped off the light and waited, afraid to breathe. Nothing happened.

Minutes later, Jennifer saw tabulated results of animal studies on printout sheets on the desk, but nothing to indicate how to operate the computer, and nothing about the human studies.

In desperation, she searched the computer itself, found the power switch. She bit at her lower lip and flipped it to the "On" position, praying it would not activate some horrific loud bell or siren as a security device. The machine hummed and whirred and came to life quietly. Jennifer took a deep breath and tentatively touched the numbers 997 on the computer's keyboard. The numbers 997 appeared on the video screen, but only stared back at her. She pressed a key marked "Prnt" and jumped back when something whirred and clacked at one side of the machine. When she looked, a printout page offered itself through a slot facing the desk. On it, she read "997." Nothing more. Jennifer typed out "Lisa Waters" on the keyboard and punched the "Prnt" key. Again, the printout sheet read only what she had typed into the machine. Damn. She tried "Laniet Teague." Nothing. She must be doing something wrong, she decided. On an impulse, Jennifer typed "Stephanie Adams," punched "Prnt". After a familiar whirring and clacking, she read:

"*Adams, Stephanie.* F. 23. Dental. IPT-4. 1-#3. PPT-8 S-0. RD-0. D-0. BP-120/80. R-20. P-84. 1063."

Jennifer searched her memory for other patient names and punched them into the computer. The results were similar. She guessed the IPT meant "initial pain tolerance," PPT the "posttreatment pain tolerance." S could mean "sedation." RD, probably "respiratory depression." D? "Depression"? "Dizziness"? "Discontinued treatment"? BP, P, and R were standard for "blood pressure," "pulse" and "respiration." And 1063 had to be the code number assigned to Steph Adams. 1-#3 must mean she had one injection of drug number three, Opain. Jennifer punched in "Arnold Heath":

"*Heath, Arnold.* M. 26. Neuro. IPT-3 1-#4. PPT-14. S-0. RD-0. D-0. BP-124/80. R-22. P-86. 943. LTF."

So Heath had been in the study. LTF had to mean "lost to follow-up," that he never returned for his follow-up visits. No wonder, Jennifer thought. He was crushed and pulverized on the Major Degan Expressway, brain tumor and all, bounced along under speeding automobiles like a blood-filled rag doll. She tried to force the picture from her mind. She typed out "Maria Ortez," but nothing happened. Frustrated at being unable to unlock the computer's secrets, Jennifer started to leave. As a last try, she typed into the keyboard the word "Opain." Just then, she heard a door slam again somewhere outside, and the computer went crazy, whirring and clacking noisily at breakneck speed, a long stream of paper gushing forth from its side, spilling over the desk and onto the floor. Jennifer grabbed for the paper as it wriggled and squirmed as though alive, tried to gather it up in her arms. The machine suddenly stopped dead silent, only the noisy crackling sound of her attempts to fold the long sheet of paper audible above her bounding pulse.

The sound of someone walking down the hall made Jennifer stop her frantic efforts and stand perfectly still. She had an overpowering urge to switch off the computer, certain it had paused only momentarily and would spin to life again any instant, giving her away. Soft footsteps approached the door where she stood. They stopped just outside. Jennifer couldn't move. A piece of the long paper scraped against her coat as her hands trembled uncontrollably. Passing seconds seemed like eons in her heightened state. At last, the footsteps moved again and passed down the hall, giving her the courage to take a much-needed breath. When a door slammed again, Jennifer switched off the computer, the light, and cracked the door to the outside hall. Empty. She quickly pulled the door shut, locked it, and raced for home, endless feet of computer printouts stuffed beneath her coat.

At home, Jennifer rolled the long printout sheets up from each end like a scroll. She sat at her desk and tried to decipher the results. She spent more than an hour just scanning the names and code numbers trying to find "Laniet Teague," "997," or "Lisa Waters." They weren't there. The results appeared very consistent with drug number three, which she knew had to be Opain. Each patient's pain threshold went up significantly. Most at least doubled. She felt a lump in her throat when she saw Kid Foster's name, and thought of the strapping young boxer lying paralyzed and helpless facedown on his tubular steel bed, waiting for someone to rotate the bed every two hours so he could stare at the ceiling instead of the floor. Dependent for life on someone else to feed him, bathe him, hose him off when his incontinent bowels and bladder chose to empty themselves. A hopeful young fighter, defeated before his main bout.

Among others, Jennifer couldn't find "Ella Lu Mavis" on the printout sheets. One pattern did emerge, though only in a few cases. Patients who received drug number four showed remarkable increase in their pain tolerance, but all seemed to receive another drug, number five, as well. Posttreatment pain tolerances seemed to revert to initial levels after number five. IPT-4. 1-#4. PPT-12. 1-#5. PPT-4. Jennifer had no idea what numbers four and five were. Maybe Neilson was already working on another drug.

At eight P.M. Jennifer called David West to tell him about the printouts.

"You what? I thought you were joking."

"I had to know, David."

"Well? Is Kane hiding bodies somewhere?"

"I can't find a thing. Arnold Heath is on the computer. Lost to follow-up."

West didn't answer right away. "Jennie, you could get in big trouble stealing those results. You better burn them."

"Don't you want to see them first?"

"I can't tonight. I'm tied up. And you shouldn't keep them around."

"Afraid of not getting your staff appointment?" she asked.

"It's not that. But I sure as hell wouldn't if they thought I helped steal research records. You know how big Opain is. Everybody in the world wants it. Neilson would crucify you."

She laughed. "I don't think so, David. Have fun with your pretty little nurse."

West grunted something unintelligible. "Sure. Say hi to Steve."

Minutes later, Jennifer shoved the scroll behind her desk to answer a knock on the door.

"Got your new lock," the superintendent said.

"It's about time."

He ignored her remark and came inside, trailing a drill cord behind. "Got a beer?"

"No."

He shrugged, set the box on the floor, and made pencil marks on the door above a ruler. Jennifer stood with arms folded, watching him work. In such a tiny room, there was no place to go. When the phone rang, she tried to hear above his whining drill.

"Wardner," the nurse shouted. "Fourteenth floor. She's hysterical with pain. Please hurry."

Jennifer grabbed her coat and ran through the cold night to the hospital. In Melanie's room, she found two nurses holding the frail girl on the bed, flapping and squealing like a tethered bird. Great heart-wrenching sobs filled the voids between her shrieks.

"She's been hurting all day," a red-faced fat nurse shouted. "Refused to take anything. Now that it's night, naturally she's changed her mind."

Jennifer tried to get Melanie's attention, ignoring the angry nurse's running condemnation. Finally she was able to wipe Melanie's sweat-drenched brow and speak during a rare instant of silence. "Let her go," she told the nurses.

"You can't let her go," the fat woman challenged. "She's hysterical. Being ridiculous."

"Let her go," Jennifer said, straightening, feeling her anger rise. "What's her blood pressure?"

"Two hundred over one-thirty," the angry nurse shouted.

"Pulse?"

"Who could take it with her like this? It was one-eighty-six an hour ago."

Jennifer felt the pressure pounding in her head. Melanie had to be near her viable pain tolerance. "Let her go," she demanded. "I'll take the responsibility." When they did, Jennifer bent over Melanie and whispered, "It's Dr. Barton, Melanie. Try to tell me about it."

The girl continued to move about restlessly in the bed, but tried to speak between her shaking sobs. "Hurts so bad," she moaned.

"Where does it hurt?"

Melanie shook her damp head, scrunched up her face. "Everything hurts."

Jennifer reached for Melanie's hand, but the girl jerked away and opened wide, frightened eyes. "It's never been this bad. Please. Help me."

Jennifer forced a smile. "I'll be right back. Try to hold on."

The fat nurse ignored Jennifer while she dialed Neilson's number from the nurses' station outside. It was busy. After several tries Jennifer asked the operator to break into the line. Melanie's anguished screams echoed down the hall, muffled only slightly when somebody closed her door.

"There's nobody on the line," the operator said. "I'll report the number out of order."

Jennifer hung up. In desperation she dialed Nurse Kane's number. Melanie had to get an injection of Opain. Kane didn't answer. Jennifer stood, told the fat nurse, "Give her fifty of Demerol now. I'll be back as soon as I can."

Outside Neilson's apartment, Jennifer asked the taxi driver to wait and raced inside. She took an empty elevator up to his floor, and ran down the carpeted hallway to his apartment door, praying he'd be home. Seconds after she rang his bell, the door opened.

"Well, hello, Jennifer," Nurse Kane said in a husky tone.

Jennifer could hardly believe her eyes. Nurse Kane stood smiling, her blond hair flowing in gentle curves across one bare shoulder above a strapless burgundy evening dress, the same color as the smeared lipstick on her thin lips.

Kane stepped back to open the door even wider, gestured toward the interior with her half-filled champagne glass. "Come in."

15

Jennifer walked quickly past Nurse Kane, to see Dr. Neilson rise from the sofa in a black velvet jacket and gray slacks. A dancing fire glowed bright yellow in the fireplace, and sounds of a mellow jazz piano floated into the room. "Well, Jennifer," Neilson said, turning on a table lamp, his voice a bit too professional. "What brings you out into the cold night? Let me get you some champagne."

Kane closed the door and returned to a corner of the sofa, pulling her stocking feet under her dress. She lit a cigarette and tried to smile at Jennifer, resting one arm on the back of the sofa where Neilson had sat.

"It's Melanie Wardner," Jennifer said. "She's in severe pain again."

Neilson looked confused. "Wardner . . . Wardner . . ."

"With the ruptured bladder. Fourteenth floor."

"Of course. I thought she was much better."

"She was. At least, regarding her pain. She's worse than ever now. And she's too weak to take much more."

Kane leaned forward toward the coffee table and poured an extra glass of champagne. "Sit down, Jennifer." She patted the seat beside her. "You may as well have something while you tell us about it." She offered the glass.

173

"I have a cab waiting. But thank you anyway." Jennifer turned to Neilson. "She really needs some Opain."

Neilson nodded, set his glass down. "I'll get it." He walked toward the rear of his apartment.

Jennifer suddenly felt like a dunce standing in the corner.

"Don't look so surprised, Jennifer," Kane said matter-of-factly. "Nurses are women, too."

Jennifer swallowed. "You look very nice."

"Thank you. Would you like one of us to go with you?"

"I can take care of it, Nurse Kane. She just needs an injection."

Kane nodded, smiled. "Rachael, please. It's after hours."

Jennifer tried to smile. Kane's perfume lingered in the air despite the cigarette smoke. Neilson reappeared before she had to speak again, handed her an unmarked glass vial. "This should do it," he said. "If there's any problem, call me."

Jennifer thanked him. "Your phone's off the hook," she said, catching Kane's quick glance toward her. "Or out of order."

"Ah, yes," Neilson said. "I have to take it off occasionally for a little peace and quiet. I'll replace the receiver."

Kane didn't stand, but nodded from the sofa when Jennifer said good night. In the elevator and in the taxi back to the hospital, Jennifer marveled at what she'd seen. Nurse Kane—or Rachael, as she preferred—was almost glamorous. Feminine. And Jennifer had no doubt either how or where she and Neilson intended to spend the remainder of the evening. Nurse Jekyll and Miss Hyde. Or vice versa.

Back on the fourteenth floor of the hospital, Jennifer quickly gave Melanie Wardner the injection of Opain. In less than twenty minutes the drained girl was fast asleep, pale and haggard, but free of pain. Jennifer recorded the injection on Melanie's chart and went home.

At home, Jennifer almost cried out when she opened the door to her apartment. Her desk drawers were all

open, their contents strewn across the floor, the sofa overturned and magazines thrown haphazardly around the
room. She listened for any sound inside before taking
her hand from the doorknob, afraid the intruder might
be hiding inside. No sound came from the bathroom or
the tiny kitchen. After a moment's consideration, she
closed the door and raced downstairs.

The superintendent made no effort to hide his annoy-
ance when he opened his door. "Now what?" he grumbled.

She told him.

His big rounded shoulders heaved a sigh of frustration.
Without speaking, he turned to get a key and long flashlight off the chrome dinette behind him and walked out
toward the elevator.

"Here," he barked as the elevator stopped on three.
He handed her a shiny key. "You forgot this. And use it
to lock your door from now on, so I can get some rest."

The superintendent barged into her apartment,
quickly confirmed that nobody was there, and left, his
face florid with anger. Jennifer said thank you to his disappearing broad back and closed and locked her door.
She tried the new lock twice, satisfied herself it was
strong and secure. She spent the next hour straightening
up the mess and trying to put things back where they
belonged. She confirmed early what she had suspected.
The computer printout sheets were gone from where she
had wedged them behind her desk. But who had known
she took them? And who would care enough to break
into her apartment and steal them back? Maybe there
was something on the sheets she had overlooked. Something that somebody was determined to keep a secret. It
couldn't be Neilson or Kane. And she'd told only David
what she'd done. But he'd have no reason to take them.
For some unknown reason, the face of the bald Chinese
man with the Vandyke beard popped into Jennifer's
memory. She dismissed it immediately. Neilson had said
he'd already shown them the results of his study. And
even given them samples of Opain to test. She ran a tub
of hot water and soaked for a long time, trying vainly to

think of anybody who might have known about the computer sheets.

A little after eleven P.M. she sipped a cup of tea and reread the letter on her desk:

> Dear Steve,
>   You always said I was determined, capable, and a little too independent for my own good. "Headstrong" was the word you used. Well, I guess you were right. I love my work and my patients and knowing I've got a profession I can do throughout my entire life. You even warned me about trying to do everything by myself. And you were right, Steve. Sometimes I'm so miserably lonely I could cry. I guess I am crying, to tell the truth. I do want the little house and the children we talked about. And a man to love. But it would take a very strong, secure man to put up with me. Like you, Steve. Good night, my darling. Sleep well. And please forgive me. I love you more than life itself.

Jennifer folded the blue stationery and dropped it into her wastebasket. After a long silent moment, she got up, rinsed out her teacup, and went to bed.

Just after midnight, the nurse on the children's orthopedic ward felt under little Juan Ortez's blanket to see if he was dry. "He's my little man," she said to her aide. "But soaking wet." She lifted Juan from his bed and cradled him to her chest while the aide stripped off the sheet from his bed, unaware of the blood dripping from beneath the blue blanket onto her uniform.

Suddenly the aide looked up, wide-eyed, and pointed. "Oh, no. Not again. Blood."

The nurse quickly shifted Juan onto one arm and looked down at the spreading red stain on her uniform. She unwrapped the blanket around Juan's feet and heard the wet splat of a blood clot hitting the floor. "Call Dr. Traymore," the nurse said. "He's ripped out his stitches again. But don't tell his poor mother. She's almost ready for the psych ward as it is." The nurse clamped her hand down near the base of the gory stub that was once Juan's big toe, slowing the pulsating spurts of crimson to a trickle as the aide ran for the phone. Raw flesh gaped open over what was left of the white bone, with only one tiny stitch remaining in place. As the nurse pressed harder against his gaping flesh, little Juan cradled his head against her breast and went to sleep.

Jennifer awoke early Saturday morning to a bright, clear day. After breakfast, she walked across the avenue to the hospital, enjoying the feel of Saturday in New York. There was an indefinable something that made it different from all the other days of the week. Maybe the traffic sounds, or the expressions on people's faces. You could tell it wasn't Sunday because everybody still walked faster than the leisurely pace typical of Sunday. Whatever, it was a beautiful morning, and she was glad to be alive.

Mr. Jennings said he was fairly comfortable, but couldn't understand why he would be in the hospital six more weeks. Jennifer tried to explain that burns heal very slowly. Jennings said he guessed he'd have to accept it, but his tone said he wouldn't.

On the fourteenth floor, Jennifer stopped short when she entered Melanie Wardner's room. She backed out to see if she had gone in the wrong room by mistake, totally confused. The room was empty, the bed stripped of all linens. And Melanie was nowhere in sight. She hurried to the nurses' station to inquire where Melanie had been transferred, and why.

"I thought you knew," the nurse said. "She died."

"What?" Jennifer held to a metal chair for support, finally had to sit down. The blood drained from her head till she thought she would faint. "No," was all she could seem to say. "No."

"Right after midnight," the nurse said, "according to the death certificate."

Jennifer stared into space, unbelieving, as the nurse

bustled around her, preparing medications and making notes on patients' charts. When she could, Jennifer asked for details.

"The night nurse said she just went to sleep. They found her after the shift change."

Jennifer picked up the phone and called Neilson's home number. He grunted something into the phone, obviously half-asleep. "Melanie Wardner's dead," Jennifer said.

Neilson came awake instantly. "When?"

She told him.

"What time did you give her the Opain?"

"About nine-forty-five, maybe ten. I came straight back here."

There was a moment's silence before Neilson spoke. "I'll be right over. Meet me in the morgue."

While Jennifer waited for Neilson to arrive outside the pathology-department offices, she answered a page on her beeper. The call was from Dr. Peterson, in Pathology. She went inside the offices and asked for him. Peterson emerged from a back office in green scrub pants and shirt and crumpled long white coat. He chewed at a stubby cigar in one corner of his mouth and looked at Jennifer over half-frame black-rimmed glasses. He motioned her inside.

"What was in that injection you gave the Wardner girl?"

"I . . . something for pain," Jennifer said.

Peterson tilted his chair back and ran his palm across the top of his head, where his hair used to be. His cigar wiggled slightly, found its place. "Doctor, pretend I'm not an idiot, okay? What the hell was in the injection?"

Jennifer sat as calmly as she could in front of his littered desk, watched him sip coffee from a Styrofoam cup. "I don't think I can tell you. Not yet."

Peterson took off his glasses with one hairy hand, rubbed his eyes with the other. "And just when can you tell me, young lady? After being up all night, I'm a little short of sleep. And patience." He put his glasses back on.

They were finger-smudged, but he didn't seem to notice. He glared over them at Jennifer.

She cleared her throat. "Dr. Neilson is on the way here. I'd rather he tell you."

Peterson put both elbows on his crowded desk, rested his stubbled chin in one hand. "Dr. Neilson, huh?"

Jennifer nodded, pressing her lips together.

"Well, while we're waiting, why don't you just tell me about Melanie Wardner. Everything you know. Maybe it'll help keep me awake."

Jennifer told Peterson about Melanie's initial problem, a small stricture in her urethra, limiting proper drainage of her bladder. And about her ruptured bladder. Everything she knew. When she finished, she fell silent while Peterson made notes and slurped his black coffee. His cigar was nauseating. She began to realize how foolish she'd been to give Melanie the injection. An unmarked vial. An unproven drug in the eyes of the law. Unlicensed by the FDA. Illegal. She could be convicted of murder. Maybe Neilson had a license to test new drugs as a research scientist. But what if he denied any knowledge of Jennifer's giving it? To protect his precious Opain. Only Nurse Kane had witnessed him giving her the vial. And there was no hope of expecting Kane to admit it. She'd support whatever Neilson said till the East River went up in flames. Jennifer's discomfort grew with each silence-breaking tick of the big round clock on the wall behind Peterson. Worst of all was the nagging doubt that maybe she had killed Melanie. Maybe the drug in the vial wasn't Opain. It could have been anything. Instead of helping that tiny, defenseless girl . . . Jennifer felt her eyes sting, took a Kleenex from her pocket to blow her nose. "All for a little pinched pee tube," Melanie had said. And now a cold slab in the morgue.

"Look, the girl died less than two hours after Dr. Barton gave her the injection," Peterson said. "How the hell can we not suspect it?"

Dr. Neilson stood to one side of Jennifer. Nurse Kane was at his side, wearing the same dress she'd had on the night before. Neilson leaned on Peterson's desk. "Opain didn't kill her," Neilson said calmly.

"You don't deny that's what Dr. Barton gave her?"

"Of course not. I gave the vial to her myself. Nurse Kane can verify it." He turned to Kane.

"It was Opain," Kane said. "I saw it."

Neilson turned back to Peterson. "You're a good pathologist, Pete. There's nobody better. But I want a neuropathologist to be with you at the autopsy. This girl suffered incredible pain from the time she came in the hospital till she died, except for when she was on Opain. I want to know what every one of her brain cells looks like. Every nerve. If Opain caused any damage at all, I have to know."

After some discussion, Peterson said he'd call in the specialist Neilson demanded, Dr. Crispin. Peterson agreed he was the best in the profession. Crispin said he could be there by noon. Neilson turned to Jennifer. "You don't have to stay, Jennifer. You look beat."

Jennifer stood, took a deep breath. "I've got to know what killed her."

Nurse Kane turned to Jennifer. "Can I get you a cup of coffee?"

"No," Jennifer said. "I think I'll go out for a breath of air. See you at noon."

The autopsy room smelled strongly of sickeningly sweet disinfectant and Peterson's cigar. Harsh fluorescent lights reflected off two shiny stainless-steel tables and the polished green vinyl floor. A constant gurgle of water flushing the trough at the edges of the steel table echoed through the cold room. Jennifer tried not to stare at Melanie Wardner's slack face or her stark-white stiff body as she was placed nude on the table. The unmistakable stench of death managed to permeate the smells of cigar and synthetic flowers of the disinfectant. Peterson and Dr. Crispin, the neuropathologist, spoke in droning monotones into recording mikes hung around their necks as they worked on what used to be Melanie Wardner. Dr. Neilson stood directly behind Crispin, often leaning for-

ward for a closer look and asking muted questions or
making suggestions. Jennifer caught herself studying ob-
jects in the sterile room: a steel mop bucket, a hanging
scale with a large round dial and fenestrated tray for
weighing organs, somebody's black lunch pail and ther-
mos on a side counter next to the microscope. She
couldn't watch when Melanie's scalp was peeled forward
and folded down over her face. Somehow, the girl
seemed much smaller than Jennifer remembered. As the
noisy electric saw cut into Melanie's skull, Jennifer
found herself staring at the fresh white dressing on the
dead girl's finger, and thought it especially sad that the
finger wouldn't have time to heal.

"Superficial hemorrhages," Dr. Crispin said, pointing
to the convoluted surface of Melanie's brain. Moments
later, he separated her glistening brain from the interior
of her skull and placed it on the scales hanging nearby.
A thick yellow goo like half-melted chicken fat dripped
from the scales. Peterson worked through a long Y-
shaped incision that opened the front of Melanie from
the base of her neck to her pelvis, glancing up briefly at
Crispin's comment. Jennifer heard a wet sucking sound
as Peterson lifted Melanie's liver out of her abdomen
with both hands. He turned it over and over as he spoke
into his Dictaphone, and set it on the dripping scales
when Crispin transferred the brain to a large glass jar
filled with clear liquid.

"What about the brain stem?" Neilson asked. "I don't
see any hemorrhages there."

"Maybe on the microscopic," Crispin said.

Jennifer wasn't unhappy that she could hardly see
from where she stood behind Neilson and Crispin. And
she knew that nothing would be definitely settled until
after the microscopic studies were done and the chemical
analyses reported from the toxicology lab. She felt very
useless, but couldn't force herself to leave. Nurse Kane
had left before the autopsy began, telling Neilson she
would call him later. Jennifer gagged when Peterson
opened Melanie's bloated intestines, releasing a whistling
rush of decaying putrid gas into the room. She swal-

lowed hard at the bile in her throat, and her eyes watered. Peterson looked up at her for an instant, pushed his glasses up on his nose with one blood-smeared rubber glove, and nodded toward the door. Jennifer didn't wait for a second suggestion. She left, lurching unsteadily, only stopping to lean against the wall outside till her dizziness had almost passed.

By the time she reached First Avenue, Jennifer could see clearly again, and the ringing in her ears had stopped. She took several deep breaths of the cold air and started across the avenue as the light changed to halt traffic.

"Hey, Jennie. Wait."

David West caught up with her on the opposite curb. He looked handsome and outdoorsy in corduroy jeans and beige turtleneck under his unbuttoned sheepskin jacket. "Aren't you freezing?" he asked.

Jennifer glanced down at her white uniform. "I hadn't noticed."

"How about lunch? My treat."

A wave of nausea pushed right up to the bottom of her throat. "No."

"Why not? You look starved. You're pale green."

"I don't want to discuss it. Okay?" She walked quickly toward Brigton House, West beside her.

"Did I do something wrong?"

She finally stopped and told him about Melanie, braced by the icy river breeze on her face.

"I'm sorry," he said. "But you can't blame yourself. She just had more than she could stand."

"That's not a very scientific diagnosis."

"Okay, irreversible shock. Cardiovascular collapse. Maybe a CVA—a massive stroke. Can we talk about it?"

Jennifer hesitated, finally agreed. West accompanied her to her apartment. Upstairs, she realized how cold she really was and put on a sweater. She went over everything she could remember about Melanie's course in the hospital. "David, she said something very peculiar a couple of days ago. No, it was yesterday. It seems like forever. Her pain was coming back, but she refused to take anything for it."

"Some people do. They don't want to get hooked."

"Not that. She said she couldn't take the medicine because she couldn't stand any more pain. That she had craved it. Wanted more."

West sat forward, elbows on his knees, and frowned. "She was confused, Jennie. She meant she craved more medicine. She was afraid of becoming addicted."

Jennifer leaned back on the sofa across from him, hugged her arms to her chest. "I don't think so." She thought for a minute. "You remember the white rat that banged his head against the cage?"

West nodded. "Sure."

"I had a big chimp do almost the same thing yesterday. He would have stimulated himself to death if I'd let him. In fact, he was furious when I pulled him out of his cage, tried to attack me. Tried, hell—he did."

"What happened?"

Jennifer waved one hand in a gesture to silence him. "Doesn't matter, let me finish. Melanie tore off the entire end of her finger after she'd had some Opain. And she ignored it, treated it like a joke. When they repaired it in surgery, she refused any anesthesia."

"So?"

"So, I think she enjoyed the pain of her injury. And the surgery. Can you imagine what it's like to feel a scalpel cut into your skin while you're wide-awake? Making an incision to open up your flesh, without even any novocaine?"

West didn't comment. His intense gaze searched her face.

"And what about your man with the brain tumor? If he wanted to commit suicide, wouldn't he take a quick, easy way out? You wouldn't lie down at the edge of an expressway and stick your legs under the cars. A witness swore that's what he did. And he was on Opain."

West's discomfort with the memory was visible. "You don't know that for sure."

"I do know it. He was on the list. The computer printout."

West's face reddened. "I told you to get rid of that. Where is it?"

Jennifer stared directly into his eyes. "I thought you might tell me."

He looked genuinely puzzled. "Now you've lost me."

She waited to see if his eyes would change. They didn't. "Somebody broke in here last night and took it." She stood, walked to the window. "David, there's something wrong with Opain. Somebody is trying to cover up something."

"Or just protect their discovery. Jennie, this drug is worth billions of dollars. You've seen the crowds protesting on TV, demanding its release. Thousands of people would gladly steal whatever's on that computer. Maybe one of them followed you."

Jennifer turned to face him, almost whispered, "You're the only person who knew I had those computer records."

He stood quickly. "For God's sake, Jennifer. That's the second time you've accused me of breaking into your apartment. If I'd wanted to see the damned records, I'd have come over when you called to tell me about them. You're going off the deep end."

She considered what he said, walked into her kitchen. She didn't really want to believe it. After a long silence she asked, "How about some tea?"

Later, West convinced Jennifer to join him for lunch. She changed into jeans and her alpaca sweater-jacket, and they walked up to Friday's to join the crowd immersed in eating, drinking mugs of beer and Bloody Marys, and arguing minor intellectual points with major emotion. Jennifer picked at her chef's salad while West ate.

"It can't be all coincidence," Jennifer said. "Your patient, Heath. Melanie. Lisa Waters disappeared. Ella Lu. And probably Laniet Teague. What if they all had a peculiar reaction to Opain? Craved pain so badly they killed themselves trying to get more?"

West drank his beer. "Out of over a thousand cases?"

"It's possible. All drugs react differently in different

people." Jennifer had to almost shout to be heard above the din of music and laughter around her.

"Look, Jennie. You're a bright girl. A good doctor. You're very much a woman. You've got everything going for you. But you're stubborn. Why get all strung out on one or two things you can't explain? Sure you're upset because a girl died. Your patient. We all are when it happens. But we're not gods. We can't save everybody, no matter how hard we try."

Jennifer sipped at her wine. It was bitter. "Okay. So I am overreacting." She forced a smile, changed the subject, and tried to change her mood. "Any word on your staff appointment?"

West wiped the corner of his mouth with his napkin. "It's all set except for the final board approval. A rubber stamp."

"That's great, David. Have you picked out an office?"

He signaled the waiter for another beer. "I'm going full-time at the university. I'll practice in the hospital neurosurgery offices. And I have a grant for surgical research."

"You deserve it. What kind of research?"

"Trying to isolate the brain's pain-regulation center. Or the major endorphin site, if there is one. If we find out where it is, maybe we can determine how it works."

Jennifer almost laughed. "Surgical Opain?"

West raised one eyebrow, smiled. "Something like that."

"Who's giving the grant? NIH?"

West shook his head, grinned. "Neilson."

"You're kidding." She saw the gleam in his eye. "You're *not* kidding."

West folded his arms on the table. "It was his idea. My chief loved it."

"So the great neurosurgeon who barely tolerates research becomes a researcher."

"Oh, no. It's only a couple of afternoons a week. The rest of the time I'm in surgery."

Jennifer studied her salad for a moment. "Is that why

you're so defensive about Opain? Because of Neilson's grant?"

West took her hand across the table. "You know better than that. If there was one ounce of evidence Opain caused problems, I'd be the first to yell about it. No, probably the second. I think Neilson would be the first. He lives and breathes finding the perfect painkiller. It's all he ever thinks about."

Jennifer thought of Nurse Kane lounging on Neilson's sofa. Of Neilson's late-night call inviting her over for a nightcap. Of the three Chinese men and the Swiss bank account. She pushed her salad bowl away and folded her napkin. "I'm glad you got your appointment, David."

West took the hint, paid the waiter, and they left. On the slow walk home, Jennifer asked, "Can you imagine what might happen if nobody in the world ever felt any pain?"

"They'd quit making aspirin."

"Be serious."

"Okay. I'm imagining."

"Maybe pain is a necessary stimulus. Like excitement. Or love. Exercise. Even sex. Any form of stimulation. If you didn't have it, you'd try to find it."

"The sex part, I go along with."

She ignored his comment. "If there's no excitement, people become very bored. They crave stimulation. Like joggers. You know they get a certain high from running. Joggers' high is probably from elevated endorphins in their systems. Why do you think so many people smoke pot? Sniff cocaine?"

"To escape reality."

"Maybe. But maybe they're just bored. Looking for a new high. A new thrill. I bet if you took all pain away from people, even the little subliminal pains we have that we're not conscious of, they'd keep trying bigger and bigger hurts till they could feel something again."

"Only the masochists. Jennie, most people can't stand even the tiniest ache. Look at the millions of over-the-counter drugs sold every year. Check the TV commercials. Stuff for headache pain, sore throat, arthritis, muscle aches, bursitis, hemorrhoids. Half the country's on Valium or Librium so they won't feel lonely or depressed, won't get upset no matter what happens in their lives. Parents are on booze or tranquilizers so they won't feel anything emotional, and kids are on uppers and downers and everything in between trying to find something that makes them feel good. To prove they're alive."

Jennifer heard him out. "Maybe. But little pains lead to a sort of pleasure too. Scratching a mosquito bite feels good. The little grumbling sensation in your stomach when you're hungry leads to satisfaction when you eat. The fullness in your bladder that feels so good when you finally get to the bathroom. Maybe not the pains themselves, but the sensation when they are relieved feels good. If you didn't have the little pains, you'd never have the little pleasures. You wouldn't appreciate them."

"But not the big hurts. Real pain."

"Maybe if you're on a drug like Opain, you can't feel those little pains. Even the big ones. Can you imagine needing to feel a little pain so badly that you keep trying bigger and bigger hurts that you still can't feel? What is the ultimate big hurt? Fire? Lying down on an expressway? A nuclear war?"

When they arrived at Jennifer's apartment building, she turned to say thanks for lunch. West insisted on walking her upstairs. At the door, Jennifer said she really had some work to do, and started inside.

West took her arm, turned her to face him. "Not even a kiss of congratulations for the new professor?"

She intended nothing more than a friendly kiss to celebrate his staff appointment, but his lips were soft and searching, and her own lips seemed to melt under their weight, opening at the first touch of his tongue. Her breath caught for a moment, and she pulled herself close against him, his hard, muscular arms encircling her till she could hardly breathe. She moaned softly when he pressed himself against her, acutely aware of the depth of her own needs. Her flesh tingled at his touch as he slipped his hand beneath her sweater, exploring her back and waist. One hand brushed lightly across her breast, then settled firmly into place and kneaded her gently, almost overpowering her mind with delicious yearnings. West pulled his face just away from hers for an instant. "My God you're beautiful," he said, lowering his lips to her neck, his breath warm, his lips hungry.

Jennifer forced her eyes open wide, took a deep breath to clear her head, and rested her hand on his. "Congratulations, professor," she said. "But this isn't getting my work done."

His dark eyes were bottomless, hungry, his jaw hard beside full soft lips. "It's about this pain I have, doctor," he whispered.

She forced herself to suppress her desire, kissed the tip of his nose, and slipped inside the doorway. "Thanks for a lovely afternoon, David. I needed it."

At about the time Jennifer carried her spun-dry clothes up from the basement laundry room, Lisa Waters slumped down unconscious in the wooden chair behind the abandoned morgue. Her head rolled to one side for an instant, then fell forward on her limp neck, unmoving, as the control button slipped from her grasp.

"Has she been up to twenty before?" Nurse Kane asked.

"Eighteen," Josef said. "This morning."

Kane flipped off the power switch, stripped a piece of graph paper from the console. "Pressure, one-seventy over a hundred. She can take more, Josef. Tomorrow morning, attach the electrodes to her teeth as well."

Josef unstrapped and lifted the tiny girl from the chair, placing her effortlessly on the bed as though she were an infant. "Her heart was irregular between nineteen and twenty," he said.

Kane pulled on her overcoat, began tying her scarf. "We have to know, Josef. It may be our last chance." She watched him secure the leather straps around Lisa's delicate ankles, turned, and left, pulling the door closed behind her.

16

At five-thirty Saturday evening, Jennifer called Melanie Wardner's roommate, Bea. When she answered, all Jennifer could say was, "I'm so sorry."

Bea's voice was thin and strained with emotion. "I still can't believe it. Not Melanie."

Jennifer hesitated, uncertain what more she could say. "She didn't suffer. Not at the end."

"She was so young. So alive. She had her whole future ahead of her," the girl whined. "What went wrong?"

Jennifer held the phone with both hands, her vision blurring. "I don't know, Bea. We'll know by the first of the week."

"Did they ... ? An autopsy?"

"Yes. They had to. The medical examiner."

Bea's voice broke completely. "It's so unreal," she sobbed. "A nightmare."

Jennifer waited, feeling the girl's agony through the phone. She wiped a tear from her cheek. "I just had to call. If I can do anything to help, please call me."

Bea said she would, and hung up.

Jennifer rinsed her face in cold water, was just drying it when somebody knocked on her door. She opened the door to see Dr. Neilson.

"May I come in?"

She showed him into her small apartment, embarrassed at the ironing board and basket of clothes near the kitchen wall. "What did they find?" she asked.

"Brain hemorrhages. Small ones, diffuse. Hemorrhage in the adrenal glands. An early ulcer in the stomach. Spotted ulcers in the colon. We'll know more Monday or Tuesday."

Jennifer nodded, asked if he'd like to sit.

Neilson sat on the sofa, frowned. "I think her pain killed her."

Jennifer sat across from him. "But she had Opain."

He nodded, still frowning. "Maybe too late. If she'd had it earlier, she'd still be alive."

Jennifer thought of Melanie writhing in her bed, struggling against her restraints, gagged and bound. "There was something very strange about the way she reacted a few days ago."

Neilson straightened on the sofa, his face querulous.

"She had to be restrained to keep from pulling out her catheter. And she ripped off the tip of her finger. Hardly noticed it. Could Opain have caused that?"

Neilson lowered his head, cleared his throat. After a long moment he looked up, concerned. "No."

Jennifer heard the slight huskiness in his voice. "Then what did?" she asked.

His voice was stronger now. "The shock of her ordeal, Jennie. She became hysterical."

"How did she get over it so quickly? One day she was like a wild animal. The next, she was so exhausted she was limp."

He leveled his gaze at her. "Maybe the autopsy will tell us." He glanced around the room. "I didn't mean to barge in on you." He stood and walked to the door. "I'm flying to Washington tonight. I'll be back on Monday."

Jennifer tried to sound cheerful. "Now who wants Opain?"

He didn't smile. "Apparently the U.S. government. I got an invitation I couldn't refuse."

Jennifer saw the concern in his eyes. "Are they going to try to stop you?"

"Maybe. But they won't."

"What will you do?"

"Whatever it takes. Move to another country if necessary."

Jennifer touched his arm. "Maybe they just want to test it. So you can release it in the States too."

Neilson tried to smile. "I hope so, Jennie. But I doubt it."

"Where would you go?"

He shrugged. "Almost anywhere I want. I've had incredible offers from all over. The Middle East, South America, Japan, Germany, France. China. I even had a call from the Russian embassy." He reached for the doorknob.

"Good luck," she said.

He took a deep breath. "Thanks."

After Neilson left, Jennifer finished her ironing and wrote a note to Kid Foster. She tore up the first two attempts, finally settled on a brief message that she hoped was cheerful and encouraging. She said she'd come to see him soon. Before bedtime, she wrote another letter:

Dear Steve,

We discussed pain before, and how you learn to live with it. But there are so many kinds of pain. How do you measure the pain of helplessly watching a vivacious young girl slowly deteriorate and die? Or the pain of her roommate's loss? How much does a dedicated young boxer suffer when he becomes paralyzed from the neck down for life? Or his fiancée, who must sit by helpless and watch him slowly give up all hope? Isn't it painful for a man to watch people shy away from him, repulsed by a face badly scarred from being burned? Or a mother whose only daughter disappears without a trace, not even saying good-bye? How much does failure hurt? Rejection? Never

knowing your parents? Being ugly, or different?
To almost win? Can it possibly hurt as much to
never know love as it does to lose it? I ache for
you, my darling Steve. And I pray your pains
may always be few and far between.

As Jennifer turned out her lights to go to bed, she saw
tiny snowflakes swirling outside her window. Hugging
her terry-cloth robe around her, she stared out the window beyond the alley to the street below, watching the
fresh snow dance beneath a streetlight. She thought of
how Melanie Wardner would have loved to walk and
laugh in the fresh snow with her friends, and tried not to
recall the picture of the hollowed-out, lifeless girl sliced
open from stem to stern on a cold steel table under impersonal white lights, her life's juices being flushed
through the table's gurgling trough into that final drain.
Jennifer heaved a great sigh and started to turn from the
window, but stopped short when something caught her
eye near the corner of the alley. A shadow had moved,
or was it her imagination? She strained to see, but all was
perfectly still. Cardboard boxes sat piled on trash cans
where a thin stream of light penetrated the dark from
the street. But nothing more. She stepped to the side of
the window, continuing to watch. Nothing. Suddenly
restless, Jennifer turned on her bedside lamp, filled a
watering pot in the kitchen, and watered her African violets on the windowsill, watching the darkness below
from the corner of one eye. She emptied the pot into the
sink, turned off the light again, and removed her robe.
Instead of going to bed, she sidled up to the window for
one last peek, just in time to see a tall figure in a heavy
coat disappear around the corner of the alley toward the
street, lurching, obviously drunk. She stood frozen, and
watched for a long while, but the man did not return. At
length, she double-checked the lock on her fire-escape
window and went to bed, lying with the blanket
huddled around her neck, eyes wide open in the dark,
staring at the frosted window, and cursing her overactive
imagination.

It was three A.M. when Jennifer's phone jangled so loudly she jumped straight up in bed. She fought to understand what the urgent voice was saying.

"Hysterical with pain, and nothing helps. We can't touch her. Hurry."

Jennifer threw on her uniform and raced through the tunnel under First Avenue toward the emergency room. Her heels echoed loudly throughout the abandoned cavern, her isolation causing her to glance nervously around each corner she passed and into each shadowed doorway. Halfway through the tunnel, the sparse overhead light bulbs flickered and dimmed. *Not now*, Jennifer begged. *Not now.* She quickened her pace, watching the dusty bare bulb ahead of her strain to stay alive, its filament a dull red glow. Water dripped steadily somewhere down a darkened side corridor, its sound reverberating off solid concrete walls in the silence. Jennifer almost screamed when a metal door suddenly scraped and jerked open in a shadow just ahead. She flattened herself against the far wall, uncertain which way to run. A burly man in khaki pants and sweater stepped from the shadows, his face round and black, his hair short and wiry, like a toupee of steel wool.

"Didn't mean to scare you," he said, pulling a mop-filled bucket into the light.

Jennifer couldn't speak. Her hands were colder than the damp wall they clung to, and shaking. Her heart was in her throat. She pushed herself from the wall and almost ran toward the hospital. When she was no more than a few steps away, the lights suddenly brightened strobe white and abruptly went out. Jennifer felt for the cold wall again and leaned against it, totally blinded in the pitch-black catacomb. Something scraped and squeaked behind her as she searched the dark with wide, straining eyes. Her heart nearly pounded through her chest.

An echoing bass voice rumbled somewhere to her right. "Damn generator," he said.

Jennifer jumped, started, when something snapped and hissed and a blinding flame assaulted her eyes. A strong smell of sulfur invaded her nostrils, and the janitor's round face gradually came into view, dancing in the match's flickering yellow glow. She let out her breath as he took a candle from his pocket and lit it, shaking out the wooden match.

"I'll lead you up the hall, doctor."

She thanked him and forced her pace to slow to his as he pulled the squeaky-wheeled mop bucket along the concrete floor of the tunnel. As they approached the elevator, the power came back on. Afraid of getting stuck in the elevator if the power went off again, Jennifer thanked him and ran up the stairs to the emergency room.

"She's absolutely wild," the emergency-room nurse said, opening the door to the treatment room.

Inside, Jennifer saw a long-legged slender girl strapped down on the exam table, her face contorted and splotched, soaked with perspiration. Her hair was a fiery orange, and she had a filthy plaster cast on her right arm.

"What's her name?" Jennifer asked, certain she already knew.

The stocky nurse shook her head. "No way to know. She just babbles when you try to talk to her. No identification."

Jennifer approached the red-haired girl, saw fresh and crusted circular burns on her arms and face. "Cigarette burns?"

"Dr. Jones thinks so. He checked her over. There's more on her abdomen and thighs. Her right big toe's broken. Looks like whip marks on her back. Big red bleeding welts all over. He put ointment on them."

Jennifer reached for the girl's hand, but she recoiled violently, screaming a bloodcurdling shriek of agony.

Jennifer saw the girl shake with heart-wrenching sobs, her eyes squeezed shut, her jaw trembling. "Vital signs?"

"Pressure one-eighty over one-twenty. Pulse two hundred."

Jennifer leaned over the girl's face, careful not to brush against her skin. "Laniet?"

The girl seemed beyond hearing. She tried again.

"Laniet? Are you Laniet Teague?" She only shook and sobbed.

Jennifer turned to the nurse. "Who brought her in?"

"She was dumped," the nurse said. "Some guy with a beard yelled 'Emergency' through the door and ran. We found her on the curb. Not even a coat."

Jennifer hurried to the phone, tried to get Neilson's number, hoping against hope he might have changed his plans. No answer. She searched her mind frantically for a solution other than calling Nurse Kane. This girl had to be Laniet Teague. She thought of calling Mrs. Teague, to be sure. The intern on duty stopped at Jennifer's side for a moment. "Her pressure's up to one-ninety," he said. "You want to treat it, or shall I?"

"What do you think it is?"

He narrowed his bloodshot young eyes. "Beats hell out of me. I gave her a hundred of Demerol. Didn't help. She must be on drugs. Maybe a withdrawal. I drew a blood sample."

Jennifer made her decision. She had no choice. "I'll take care of it," she said, picking up the phone.

Minutes later, Nurse Kane said, "Meet me in the clinic. We'll admit her to the second floor."

Jennifer helped transfer the shrieking girl to a stretcher, and accompanied her to the Pain Control Clinic. The orderly left her alone with her patient, now reduced to a quivering mass of splotchy flesh and wet sobs, still incoherent. Jennifer had not told Kane who she thought the girl was. She just hoped her patient didn't die before Opain had a chance to work. And she wanted to watch Kane's face when she saw Laniet Teague.

Kane arrived at a half-trot, glanced at the girl with no hint of recognition, and unlocked the door to the lab. Moments later, she emerged with a loaded syringe in hand and gave the resisting girl the injection in her thigh. She asked about her pressure and pulse. Jennifer told her.

"I'll admit her, Jennifer. You get some sleep."

"I'll stay," Jennifer said. "I'm already awake."

Kane glanced at Jennifer, back to the girl. "Whatever you like." She began to turn the stretcher toward the corridor.

Jennifer helped push the stretcher to the elevators, pressed the button for the second floor. "Is this girl a patient of the clinic?" Jennifer asked.

"No."

Jennifer moved to one side of the stretcher, watching Kane's face. "You're sure it isn't Laniet Teague? Number 997?"

Kane stood impassive. "I have no idea who she is. I never saw her before."

Jennifer persisted. "You remember the woman who came by looking for her daughter? A redhead with a broken arm?"

The elevator doors opened on two. "Oh, yes," Kane said. "The alcoholic woman." She pulled the stretcher from the elevator. The patient seemed calmer already, lay perfectly still, but her face was still contorted.

"The description fits," Jennifer said. "I think this is Laniet Teague."

"Maybe it is," Kane said. "Ask her in the morning."

Jennifer pushed in silence as they approached the ward. "Maybe I should call her mother, have her come down here. She'd want to know."

Kane turned as they approached the nurses' station. "That's a good idea, Jennifer." She smiled. "Why don't you have her come by first thing in the morning? After this poor child has some rest."

Jennifer had to search to find the night nurse on the ward. There were only two patients in the beds, both asleep. The other six beds were empty. Jennifer finally found the nurse, a dumpy round woman of about fifty, smoking a cigarette and reading a movie magazine in a small room off the rear of the ward. She looked the type who'd given her patients an extra sleeping pill and settled down for the night. Jennifer watched her strain to force her pudgy feet into her unlaced shoes.

"Should have called ahead," the nurse grumbled. "It'll take twenty minutes to get a chart put together."

Jennifer thought she smelled gin on the woman's breath. "I'll want vital signs every fifteen minutes till her pressure's down and stable," Jennifer said as the woman waddled alongside her, chewing at something in her mouth.

"She ought to be in intensive care."

Jennifer forced herself not to react. "Call me if her pressure isn't down to normal in an hour. I'll leave my number."

Jennifer helped transfer the patient to the bed nearest the nurses' station, checked her pressure. One-thirty over ninety. Pulse one-twenty-four. The girl didn't object to being moved, or being touched, but she was still incoherent, only moaning in response to Jennifer's questions. She opened her reddened eyes once, glared wildly toward Jennifer and Nurse Kane, and immediately squeezed them shut again.

Jennifer wrote her findings on the chart. Nurse Kane touched Jennifer's shoulder. "I'm glad you called me. If there's any problem, let me know. I'll be at home." She smiled and left.

Jennifer checked on the girl once more after completing the chart. She was sound asleep, curled up on her side like a fetus, her breathing deep and regular. Jennifer told the bleary-eyed nurse she'd be at home, and wrote down her number. The nurse grunted something and stuffed it in her uniform pocket.

Jennifer had just fallen asleep a little after five in the morning when the phone jerked her awake again. She was dreaming that she was wide-awake on an autopsy table, with a cast on both arms, and Nurse Kane was lifting out her liver with long black bloody gloves, ignoring Jennifer's frantic but voiceless efforts to tell her she was still alive. She sat up and shook her head, disoriented, and reached for the phone.

"I looked everywhere," the grumpy nurse said. "She's gone."

"When?"

"Twenty, thirty minutes. I went to the bathroom, and

when I came back, she had disappeared. You'll have to sign out her chart before I go off duty."

Jennifer splashed cold water on her face, threw on her uniform dress and coat, and raced across a snow-covered and silent First Avenue. She checked the halls, bathrooms, and other patient rooms on the second floor. On an impulse, she dialed Nurse Kane's home number. Kane answered in a sleepy voice on the second ring. Jennifer hung up. "What about her clothes?" Jennifer asked. "Her dress?"

"Still here. She musta walked out in her hospital gown."

Jennifer sat at the desk for a long moment, head in her hands, dejected.

"I've had 'em sneak out before," the nurse said, sitting heavily beside Jennifer. "Mostly come in to get drugs. They don't want to pay, so they leave in the middle of the night."

Jennifer wanted to think undisturbed, but the nurse rattled on about her experiences, wide-awake now that dawn was showing itself through the east windows, cleaning up her desk in preparation for going off duty.

Jennifer left the chart on the desk and hurried to the emergency room, asked if anyone had seen her patient pass through there. Nobody had. She searched several floors, checked the streets outside. Nothing. As a final effort, she went back to the pain clinic, checked the benches and the corridors toward the lab. There was no sign of the red-haired girl anywhere. Jennifer glanced at her watch. Six A.M., Sunday. Frustrated and tired, she pulled on her London Fog, took her scarf from her pocket, and tied it around her head. As she turned to leave the clinic, something clicked behind her, like a metal door latch.

"Who's there?" she called out. "Laniet?" She ran down the hall to the door beyond the lab where she thought the sound had come from. "Laniet? Are you in there?"

When nobody answered, she banged on the door with her fists and called out again. She tried several times, but got no response. Remembering Josef's keys, she searched through her pockets, found and extracted her own key ring, but realized the other keys were in her shoulder bag at home. Finally she gave up and went home, convinced she had only heard a door rattle from an air current, a result of the increasing wind outside.

Jennifer collapsed into bed at six-thirty, and slept until David West called at noon. She fumbled for the phone and tried to speak.

"How about brunch?" West said. "There's a great little English pub down on Thirty-fourth Street."

"I can't, David. I'm really beat."

"Fine. Pick you up in half an hour." He hung up.

Jennifer managed to put the receiver back in its cradle, turned over, and went back to sleep. Thirty minutes later, she dragged herself out of bed to see who was pounding on her door.

"I love your outfit," West said.

Jennifer blinked, suddenly realized she was standing at the door in her flimsiest nightgown. She came awake immediately, wheeled around, and grabbed for her robe. "What are you doing here?"

West came inside, grinning. "I think I just forgot," he said.

Jennifer protested, but he insisted she join him for brunch. At last, he turned her toward the bathroom, smacked her on the bottom, and said, "It's too beautiful a day to miss. The whole city's white. Get dressed."

Once outside, Jennifer was happy he had forced her out of her cocoon. It was a glorious, frosty-bright day, with invigorating new air to cleanse her lungs, and the English pub was cozy and warm. They sat near an enormous stone fireplace with its black iron kettle and pot hanging at the ready by the fire, dark rich wood paneling absorbing the glare from the snow outside. David sipped ale from a pewter mug while Jennifer tasted her burgundy. She waited until after they ordered to tell him of her experience during the early-morning hours.

"It was Laniet Teague, David. It had to be."

"Jennie, do you attract weird patients, or do you have to go search for them?"

"She's the third one who's disappeared. Maybe the fourth." She told him she hadn't been able to reach Maria Ortez either.

West tilted back in his chair for a moment, came down. "It is a little strange," he said. "But it doesn't make sense."

"It has to be something connected with Opain."

West took a deep breath, exhaled slowly. "Maybe we'd better talk to Neilson."

"Then you agree with me?"

His jaw set firmly. "I think we should know more. I don't like to jump to conclusions."

Jennifer reached across the table for his hand. "Thank you, David. For believing me."

He smiled. "Jennie, I'd believe anything you said. Even if you were wrong."

Jennifer relaxed, happier than she had been in weeks, and listened to David tell her about his most challenging operations as they ate. Both her shepherd's pie and his steak-and-kidney pudding she tasted were divine. But she was fascinated with the intensity of his flashing black eyes as he described dissecting so very carefully around a life-threatening aneurysm, a weak, bulging spot in a major artery in the brain of a twenty-four-year-old man. And how he sealed it off with little silver clips just as it started to leak. His eyes misted when he told her about a beautiful four-year-old girl with a brain full of malignancy, impossible to remove. He quickly changed the subject to another success, and enthusiastically described an emergency decompression of a depressed skull fracture on a child whose metal swing had tipped over, the heavy top bar hitting her in the head.

"You love it, don't you?" Jennifer said.

He sat back in his chair, grinned. "Yeah. Hey, I didn't mean to bore you. Tell me about you. What do you want more than anything else?"

She hesitated, studied his dark angular face. "Promise you won't jump up and run out laughing?"

"Promise."

She sipped her wine, set it back on the oak table. "A home."

She watched his eyes dilate slightly, full of warmth. "I'd never laugh about that."

She studied the table, looked up. "I also love my work. The surgery. Rebuilding people. But I never had a home, either. Not really. I don't know if it's possible, but I want both."

West leaned forward, his voice soft. "And Steve?"

Jennifer chewed at a corner of her lip, made her decision. West's eyes were sympathetic, understanding. "Steve is dead," she said, aware of the huskiness in her voice.

West didn't speak. He waited.

"He died two years ago. It wasn't very pleasant." She blinked several times, rapidly, to stop the tears from overflowing. "I'm sorry," she said, looking around the room at copper plates on the wall, a dartboard, hanging mugs, until she could continue. "He was a concert pianist. He developed a strange type of degeneration of the spinal cord. It wasn't M.S., it wasn't anything anybody could give a name. But it just got worse and worse." She sniffed, took a deep breath. She hadn't wanted to tell him. It was too personal to share. But, having started, she couldn't stop it from coming out, as though a dam deep inside her had burst, and her very core was gushing out. "He was in constant pain for the whole last year. But he hated to admit it to me. He lost the use of his hands first, then his legs. He could hardly move his head. But he always told me how beautiful life had been. How beautiful it could be, if you stopped to look."

West waited patiently while Jennifer took a Kleenex from her bag and blew her nose. "Go on," he said. "He sounds like a hell of a guy."

She nodded. "Toward the end, all he could do was read or listen to music. Sometimes I'd read to him. But he loved to try to do it himself. To prove he could. I'd watch him lie there, skin and bones, his nerves raw, in horrible pain, his mind fully alert, trying to turn the pages with that twisted claw he had left for a hand. Oh, God, David, I prayed for him to die. I needed him so much, but I used to lie awake at night and think about giving him an overdose of morphine. I couldn't stand to watch him suffer so." When West didn't interrupt, she had to continue. "I could have put an end to his suffering, David. But I didn't. I let him down when he needed me most. I watched him lie there in pain. Drenched in his own sweat and fighting to keep from crying out." She had to stop for a long moment, her eyes squeezed shut. Finally she could say it. "I failed the man I loved, David. I'm a doctor, and I couldn't help him." She sobbed out loud. "I'm afraid to ever have to make that decision again. I couldn't do what I knew had to be done. I don't ever want to fail anybody else."

After a long silence, while Jennifer tried to regain her composure, West spoke. "And you felt guilty when you couldn't."

She nodded, brushing the tears from her cheeks.

"Jennie. If you had, you could never live with yourself." He waited. "Sometimes it takes more strength *not* to do something than to do it."

She shook her head, unable to speak.

West hesitated, then asked, "Did he ask you to kill him?"

She tried to stop it from coming out. But it was no use. "Yes," she almost shouted. "Yes, dammit, yes. And I couldn't do it. I wasn't even with him when he died." Jennifer sprang up from the table and blindly ran toward the rest room, where she sat on top of the toilet and cried it out. Finally she was able to rinse her face and return to the table, spent, but somehow lightened, almost able to see herself in perspective.

"I'm sorry," she said to David. "That wasn't fair to you."

He took her hand in his. "For what it's worth, I couldn't have done it either." He smiled warmly. "You're a gutsy lady, Jennie. And one helluva fine doctor."

The waiter came, asked if they'd like another drink.

Jennifer shook her head, avoiding his eyes. "I'd like to take a walk."

Outside, Jennifer regained her control as they walked together in the snow, watching overbundled children ride on new red sleds pulled by their parents along the sidewalk. Somehow the air seemed cleaner, fresher than she remembered. One rosy-cheeked bundle threw a snowball at them from a doorway. On impulse, Jennifer scooped up a handful of snow from a parked car, balled it carefully, and winked at West. The child's giggles came from just around the brick corner, but Jennifer waited until his patience ran out and he had to peek. She tossed the snowball at the wall above his head amid squeals of joy, and she and David ran up the sidewalk, feigning great fear, before he could re-arm.

At her apartment door, Jennifer asked David if he'd like a glass of wine. He didn't answer, but opened the door widely, came in, and locked both locks behind them. Jennifer dusted snow off her coat and hung it up. When she turned to take West's coat, it was tossed over a chair. He stood staring at her as he unbuttoned his shirt from top to bottom.

"What are you doing?"

"You offered me a glass of wine. I like to be comfortable when I drink." He removed his shirt, tossed it on top of his coat and sweater, and began undoing his belt.

"David."

"I prefer Moselle," he said. "Or Chablis, if it's good." He unzipped his trousers and stepped out of them, adding them to the pile. He sat, wearing shorts and T-shirt, and slowly removed his shoes and socks. "Chilled, please."

Jennifer couldn't believe what he was doing. "That's enough," she said. "No more."

West seemed not to hear. He stripped off his T-shirt and walked toward her unmade bed. "You have the Sunday *Times*?" He pulled back the covers and crawled in, looking up as if surprised. "Well? Where's my wine?"

When Jennifer still didn't speak or move, West extended one hand toward her. "It's time to go on with living, Jennie. But it's your decision."

Jennifer stood speechless for several moments. Then, without a word, she stared directly back at West and pulled her wool sweater over her head, tossed it on top of his clothes. Her beige slacks came off next, after she'd kicked off her boots. West looked smug and bemused, but didn't speak. She almost balked when she reached around to unsnap her brassiere, but stripped it off and dropped it as nonchalantly as possible on the pile of clothes beside her. She took a deep breath, skinned out of her panties, and holding his gaze, walked to the kitchen and took a bottle of Moselle from the refrigerator. She set the wine, two glasses, and a corkscrew on the table beside West, forcing her face to show no emotion while she watched a wide smile spread across his face. She walked slowly around the bed and pulled back the covers. "If you want to read the paper," she said, "you'd better go home *now*. It's your last chance." And she climbed into bed beside him, almost leaping into his arms.

17

Jennifer awoke as dawn seeped through her window, the new day rapidly brightening from the fat snowflakes falling outside. She felt marvelous. Totally relaxed, contented. A slight soreness of her muscles brought back the memory of their lovemaking the evening and night before. The delicious tingling in remote parts of her body caused her to turn and watch David West's sleeping face, his beard coarse and stubbly, a coal-black comma of hair punctuating his fine forehead. She remembered the urgency of their first coupling, and was surprised at the intensity of her own response. She thought of the incredible sensations as he teased her afterward, exploring her body with eyes, hands, and lips, raising her to unbelievable heights of passion and letting her ease down slowly, carefully, only to take her back up again, higher and higher until she thought she'd surely explode. And his straining, clenching face as he pounded into her, carrying her along in his frenzy to dizzying heights she'd never thought possible, until she could no longer contain herself, and screamed out with a wild joy as her body shuddered again and again in an unending series of explosive releases. David had been tender and gentle one minute, demanding the next, then gentle again, touching, tasting, teasing, murmuring love sounds under his breath, learning and adjusting to her needs, her responses, her hungers. She felt herself dampen again with the memory of that final hour before they slept. The long, slow elliptical rhythm they drifted into, moving in unison as though they had been together through the centuries, and were one, inseparable, each only a half of the perfect union.

Jennifer turned to stare at the ceiling, amazed at her lack of guilt when she thought of the times she and Steve were together so very long ago. Whereas Steve had loved her, caressed and fulfilled her so tenderly, David had possessed her. Her mind. Her body. Her very soul. West had changed her forever. He had released something from her primal depths that she never knew existed. And it felt just great. She inhaled a great lungful of air and turned to West, brushing the strands of hair off his forehead. "Hey, professor."

West opened one flashing black eye, grinned. "You're insatiable," he said.

She kissed him lightly on the mouth, rolled over, and jumped out of bed. "And you're going to be late for work. Coffee?"

Jennifer boiled water for his instant coffee while he dressed, fixed herself a cup of tea. "David, have you ever been in the rooms behind the lab?"

"Next to the old morgue?"

"Yes."

He said he hadn't. "Why?"

She poured the hot water, handed him his cup. "I'm sure I heard somebody lock a door back there when I was looking for Laniet Teague."

"Maybe Josef. I've seen him come and go from that direction."

She thought for a moment. "I don't think so. I called out, even knocked on the door. Josef would've answered."

"Maybe Kane, then. Or Neilson."

Jennifer shook her head. "Kane was home. I checked. And Neilson's in Washington."

West shrugged, glanced at his watch. "Probably your overactive imagination. I've got to run."

"I have keys to the doors."

West pulled on his coat. "Oh, no," he said. "Don't you dare."

She straightened his collar. "Why not?"

"Because that's breaking and entering. They probably have supplies stored there. Maybe Opain. Neilson would be furious."

She nodded, stretched up to kiss his lips lightly.

West pulled her close, tilted her face up toward his. "You are something else, beautiful woman. Fantastic."

She hugged him tight, heard the slow steady beat of his heart, felt his athletic body against hers. "Thanks."

West stood back, opened the door. "Better put the wine back in the refrigerator. I like it chilled."

When he disappeared down the hall, Jennifer turned and picked up the unopened bottle of wine from the bedside table, carried it to the kitchen, and smiled to herself. It was going to be a glorious day.

"Your baby doesn't seem to feel pain," Dr. Traymore said in his high voice.

"Everybody feel pain," Maria Ortez responded, getting up from the sofa in the hospital lounge.

Traymore creased his narrow face even further. "I've called the pain clinic. The nurse is on her way up to talk to you before you leave. Did they tell you what was in the medicine you got right before you delivered?"

Maria shook her head. "No. Es my Juan gonna be okay?"

"He'll be fine, Maria. I put a little cast on his foot to protect it. You bring him back in a week."

Maria said she would, went to the ladies' room to freshen up, and sat to wait for the nurse.

When Jennifer arrived at the pain clinic that morning, Nurse Kane was nowhere around. The clinic was unlocked, and several patients sat on the benches near Kane's desk. Jennifer called the patients in one at a time and examined them. When Kane showed up thirty minutes later, two patients were through with the examination and waiting for something for their pain. Nurse Kane was as cold and professional as ever, though she did smile briefly at Jennifer when she first entered the clinic. During a lull at midmorning, Jennifer asked if Dr. Neilson had returned.

Kane's eyes hardened. "He called from Washington. He'll be back tomorrow or Wednesday."

"Problems?" Jennifer asked.

"Nothing we can't handle." Kane turned and walked down the hall toward the lab.

Jennifer saw the last of her patients and went to lunch. As she started through the cafeteria line, she searched the large room for David West. Her heart dropped when she saw him sitting with the pretty brunette nurse, his face intense as he leaned forward across the table while she spoke. Jennifer quickly turned her attention to the tuna salad and cottage cheese on the glass racks. How could he? she thought. Her vision blurred for a moment as tears filled her eyes, but she forced them back. Obviously their night together, which had meant so much to her, meant little or nothing to him. She paid at the cashier and took the first seat she could find facing away from West and his attentive nurse.

Jennifer ate quickly, leaving most of the food on her plate, and returned to the lab. Her depression deepened when she saw the large chimp sitting in a corner of his cage, head cocked to one side watching her, obviously set up for another experiment. To her surprise, the chimp appeared perfectly calm. Normal. The wild fury she had seen before was gone from his eyes. He sat calmly and picked at something in his hairy chest, then ate it. The rear door of the lab slammed, and Josef walked in.

"I won't repeat that experiment," Jennifer said. "Where's Nurse Kane?"

Josef studied her for a moment, expressionless. "Just check his pain threshold." He paused. "That's what Nurse Kane said."

"What other experiments are there?"

"That's all. When you finish, you can go home." He turned and left, locking the rear door behind him.

Jennifer found the chimp's pain threshold to be perfectly normal. She wrote it in the lab book and went for her coat. On her way out, she stopped and walked back down the hall toward the doors behind the lab, apparently leading to the old morgue. She pressed her ear to each door, heard nothing. She fought the temptation to unlock the doors and look inside. But Josef might come out any moment. Or Kane. She slung her bag over her shoulder and left.

As Jennifer was leaving the hospital, Nurse Kane spoke harshly into the phone at a small desk behind the animal lab. "They can't do that," she said.

"I'm afraid they can," Neilson replied. "They've canceled my patents."

"On Opain or Antopain?"

"Opain."

"But only in the U.S.?" Kane said.

"Yes."

Kane sat silent for a moment. "All right. They can't cancel patents outside the U.S. There's still a way to make them back off."

"How?"

"Not over the phone. But they'll be damned sorry they interfered."

"Rachael, it's over. At least in the States."

"You gave up too fast last time, Frank. I won't let it happen again. The big money's in this country. We'll make them pay for Antopain."

"But Antopain's worthless without Opain. It's a specific antagonist. It does nothing on its own."

"Exactly," Kane said. "And it's about to become the most valuable drug ever discovered. Call me when you get home."

When Kane hung up, she unlocked a metal cabinet beside her desk and removed a five-gallon plastic jug filled with a clear liquid. She ripped off the adhesive-tape label, identifying the liquid only as number three, and tossed it into a trash can. When the door opened, she draped her coat over the jug of Opain and turned to face Josef. "How's the woman reacting?" she asked.

"Passed out at twenty-four."

"And the baby?"

"No reaction at all up to thirty-six."

Kane thought for a moment. "Take him on up. The limit. It's got to break through somewhere."

Josef hesitated. "He's just a baby."

Kane's anger flared. "Dammit, Josef, don't you dare question me." She grabbed up her coat and the plastic jug and stormed out of the room, leaving Josef standing behind, glaring at the open door, his fists working at his sides.

Jennifer answered her beeper call at four-thirty that afternoon, returned the call to the pathology offices, and asked for Dr. Peterson.

"I've tried to get Neilson all afternoon," Peterson said.

Jennifer said he was still out of town.

"Crispin called about the findings on the Wardner girl. Looks like Neilson was right."

Jennifer asked him to explain.

"He says her nerve cells looked like they'd been fried. Brain and spinal cord. Hemorrhage and cell fragmentation in all the pain circuits. Just disintegrated."

"What about toxicology?" Jennifer asked.

"No trace of anything unusual. Only a little Demerol. What the hell's in Opain?"

"I don't know."

"Well, we couldn't find anything. If it was in her, it didn't show up."

Jennifer thanked him, said she'd tell Neilson when she saw him.

"She must have had incredible pain," Peterson said. "I've seen stress hemorrhages in the adrenals, ulcers. But never anything like this."

Jennifer hung up and walked to her window, stared out at the cold gray afternoon's fading light. The earlier snow had turned to sleet, melting the clean whiteness to sooty-black ice water splashing under the feet of over-coated New Yorkers who trudged by, huddled under their black umbrellas like mourners at a winter funeral. Jennifer shuddered at the thought of Melanie Wardner being lowered into the icy ground, unattended except for a roommate. No family. Nobody she really loved. She determined to go to Melanie's funeral, if only to comfort Bea. It was no good to be alone. It hurt too much.

Jennifer waited until six o'clock before leaving her apartment. She wanted to be sure nobody would be around the clinic or lab. She hurried through the tunnel to the hospital, passing small groups of blue-uniformed student nurses coming in the opposite direction, their laughs and cheerful conversations echoing through the dank Gothic passage—like girl scouts exploring a mountain cave. Despite their youthful faces, a few had already developed that heavy-footed walk which characterized seasoned nurses who stood on hard hospital floors at least eight hours every day.

As Jennifer had hoped, the clinic was silent, deserted. She tiptoed down the hall behind the lab, fingering the keys in her shoulder bag. She paused to listen at each of the doors, but heard nothing from inside. Reassured, she spread the assortment of keys in one palm, and tried them in succession in the lock of the last door at the end of the hall. Just as she found the one which turned the lock, she heard a muffled distant scream beyond. She froze rigid, holding her breath, her heart suddenly hammering at her ears. Only silence followed the brief out-cry, but Jennifer could swear it had been Maria's voice she heard. She tested the doorknob, carefully turning it in her palm, and winced when the metal door scraped noisily against its frame, beginning to open. Her heart nearly stopped when a door slammed with a loud bang somewhere beyond, and quick footsteps ran toward where she stood.

Jennifer pulled the door to and ran, thrusting the key into her pocket as she skidded around a corner and down the stairs toward the tunnel. Heavy footsteps ran behind her as she bounded down the concrete stairs, grabbing at the handrail to help propel her around each bend. She slammed into the door leading to the tunnel, banged it against the wall as she shot through. No more than twenty yards farther, she heard the door bang into the wall again, and heard running feet close the distance behind her. Her breath came in great gasps, her system flooded with adrenaline, but she dared not look back, thinking only of getting away. She searched desperately for help as she flew past each intersecting tunnel, but there was nobody there. She was alone. She thought at first she was losing consciousness when the lights suddenly dimmed, but she drove her aching legs faster, praying the generator wouldn't go out. She felt the heel of one shoe give way as she rounded a bend in the dim tunnel, causing her to lose her balance and rebound off the hard wet wall, limping furiously but struggling to escape. She heard panting grunts of effort from the looming shadow closing on her as she careened off the wall at the next bend in the tunnel, and saw the lights suddenly brighten white-hot and instantly go black, leaving her blinded and helpless, half-sobbing, groping along the cold sweating wall toward home. Something thudded heavily behind her, stopping the pursuit for an instant, but heavy wheezing breaths and grunts started up almost immediately. Jennifer screamed out when she ran headlong into a warm body, and fought to keep her balance as viselike hands grabbed her arms.

"Watch out, lady," a bass voice rumbled in her ear. "You can't run in the dark."

Something held her arm painfully as a match flared, and she saw the round black face of the janitor who had led her through the tunnel once before. Jennifer threw herself against his chest, clinging to him. "Somebody . . . chasing me," she gasped. "Help me."

She turned him loose when he struggled to take a candle from his pocket and lit it, peering into the darkness beyond with wide round eyes. "Ain't nobody there, doctor. Come on, I'll take you home."

Back in her apartment, Jennifer double-locked her door and sat huddled on the sofa for a long while, her heart beginning to slow. She tried to look out her window at the alley below, but the sleeting rain on the glass made it impossible to see. She tried David West's number. He wasn't in. Neilson's answering service said he was out of town. Jennifer paced the floor until after nine, asking herself again and again if she was certain what she'd heard. There was no doubt in her mind. It was Maria Ortez who had screamed. That same piercing, agonized scream Jennifer had heard in the labor room before Juan was born. But it had stopped too abruptly. Cut off, as if by a falling guillotine. Jennifer decided to confront Nurse Kane with her suspicions. She had to know. And she had to get Maria out of there. Whatever was happening had to be bad. And very painful. Jennifer tried Kane's number three times, her anguish growing with each unanswered attempt. At ten-fifteen she slammed the phone down and grabbed her London Fog and scarf, slung her bag over her shoulder, and bolted out the door.

At about the time Jennifer raced through the sleet toward New Hope Hospital, Nurse Kane lowered herself from the top of the fence in Central Park, crouching beside the five-gallon plastic jug while she watched, listened. She heard only the sound of icy rain falling on the jogging track across the fence and into the water behind her. She pulled the hood of her raincoat tighter around her face and carried the jug of Opain to the water's edge. Working quickly, she unscrewed the cap and hoisted the heavy jug with both hands.

"Hands up, bitch. Give."

Kane whirled to see two young toughs, no more than eighteen, a knife in each of their hands. The taller one grabbed the jug from her hands, tasted it. "Shit, man. It's water." He threw the jug into a nearby bush, its contents gurgling out onto the ground.

The other man crowded closer. "What's in the purse, bitch?"

"Money," Kane said. "I have money."

He grinned. "You better."

Kane fumbled with the leather bag over her shoulder. "Don't hurt me. I'll give you the money." She felt for the hard cold metal in her purse with shaky fingers, found it. "Drop the knives," she ordered, pulling a twenty-five-caliber Colt from her purse, pointing it directly at the nearest man's chest.

They immediately began to back off, slowly at first, then scrambled up and over the reservoir fence and ran. Kane quickly retrieved the plastic jug. Empty. Furious, she tossed it over the fence, hoisted herself up and over behind it. With heels sinking into the mud of the jogging track around the New York City reservoir, she marched back toward her car.

It was ten-thirty when Jennifer knocked boldly on the doors behind the lab. Nobody answered. At the most distant door, she banged loudly. Nothing. She mustered her courage, took a deep breath, and unlocked the door, ignoring its loud metallic scrape as she pushed it open and stared down the unlighted corridor. She removed her scarf, put it in her coat pocket, and fumbled for a light switch. When she switched the lights on, she saw a long hallway with several closed doors on each side. "Maria," she called out. There was no answer. She walked quickly to the first door, tried the handle. To her surprise, it wasn't locked. She flipped on the light inside and saw a standard hospital bed, empty, its mattress sagging and stained. The second room was the same. And the third and fourth. Only one door remained closed, but although there was no lock visible on her side, it wouldn't budge. Frustrated and angry, Jennifer hurried to the outside corridor and unlocked the next door behind the lab. A suffocating stench of rodents assaulted her nostrils as she opened the door, and the sounds of hundreds of fast little feet scraped against the bottoms of metal cages, then stopped all at once, lending an eerie silence to the darkened room, as though a thousand animal eyes watched, waiting for her to invade their jungle.

She stepped back into the hall, took the new book of matches from her bag, and used a lighted match to locate the light switch inside.

The room was larger than she expected, and was filled with rows of cages stacked on metal shelves along two walls. Against the third wall were eight large cages with vertical bars, empty, but apparently built to hold very large chimps. Four smaller cages sat top them, with inquisitive chimps staring silently back at her. Jennifer walked slowly through the room toward a desk in the far corner. The desktop was uncluttered, only a pencil box and phone in view. She opened the top drawer, saw a vinyl-faced notebook and glass vial labeled "Opain" in bright blue letters. She put them on the desktop and opened the book. Her breath caught when she saw the top of the first page: "Laniet Teague," was printed in bold, artistic script. Columns of dates and numbers appeared beneath, the numbers starting with 4 and gradually going up to 29. Jennifer quickly turned to the next page. "Lisa Waters." She had to sit quickly, feeling her knees give away. Similar dates and numbers filled the column beneath Lisa's name. "Ella Lu Mavis" came next, the column shorter, but the numbers higher, going to 37. If they represented levels of pain tolerated, as she suspected, Ella Lu had been subjected to a pain more than twice as excruciating as a red-hot tooth abscess, five points higher than passing a kidney stone. The next page had Maria Ortez's name on it, but no numbers. The next was for Juan Ortez. Jennifer felt something sting her right eye, and only realized it was a cold sweat dripping from her forehead when she reached to wipe it. She slammed the book closed and jumped up from the desk, tucking the book under her arm and putting the vial into her coat pocket. She had to find them. As she wheeled around to leave, she stifled a scream, and stared directly at Nurse Kane, standing in the doorway, dripping wet and muddy, pointing a gun at Jennifer's stomach.

18

"Put it back on the desk," Kane said in a tone as cold as the sleet outside.

Jennifer bristled. "Where are they?"

"Turn around," Kane said, advancing slowly toward Jennifer. When Jennifer hesitated, Kane smiled a mirthless smile, like the grin of a skull without flesh. "I won't hesitate to shoot."

Jennifer clenched her teeth, turned around. "What have you done with them? Laniet Teague, Lisa. All of them."

Kane prodded Jennifer forward with the gun in her back. At the far wall, Kane slid a rack of animal cages to one side, exposing a door Jennifer hadn't seen. She unlocked it with one hand, holding the gun to Jennifer's ribs with the other.

Inside, Jennifer almost fainted at what she saw. Little waifish Lisa Waters sat strapped into a large wooden chair, grunting, her eyes bulging, blood dripping from her lips, frantically mashing a plastic button in her right hand. Wires ran from her fingers, toes, and mouth. Jennifer saw two of the wires attached to stubs of Lisa's front teeth, drilled down to the quick. Strapped in the chair beside her, Laniet Teague panted like a wild animal, her face splotched white and red, her eyes squeezed

216

shut, and the skin on the arm where her cast had been, purple and yellow with bruises. Jennifer sank back against the door frame, shaking her head to clear her mind. Ella Lu Mavis lay facedown on a vinyl table, silent, unmoving, a clear plastic cylinder covering the length of her exposed spine.

"Keep moving," Kane ordered, shoving her ahead.

Jennifer half-stumbled to the table beside Ella Lu. The central segment of bone had been neatly cut away from each of Ella Lu's vertebrae, exposing the glistening gray tissue of her spinal cord from her scrawny neck to her coccyx. Each connecting nerve had been expertly dissected away from the surrounding ivory-white bone and had a tiny wire attached by a little silver clip. The black skin of the girl's back had been carefully sewn to the edges of the clear plastic.

"That's cerebrospinal fluid in the chamber," Kane said. "So the nerve cells stay alive. We want to be sure she feels the pain stimuli."

Jennifer turned on her. "You animal."

Kane shoved the muzzle of the gun under Jennifer's chin. "Keep calm, Jennifer."

Jennifer allowed herself to be guided through an archway into the open morgue. Beside a two-tiered bank of closed steel doors which had to house racks for corpses, Maria Ortez lay strapped to a steel table, apparently sleeping. "Maria," Jennifer called. She didn't respond.

"She's out for the night," Kane said. "You can visit tomorrow."

"Where's Juan? Her baby?"

Kane stood unblinking. "You're too curious for your own good. It's late and I'm very tired. Lie down." She nodded toward the table beside Maria.

"What are you going to do?"

"Keep you secure while I go home and get some sleep."

Jennifer reluctantly climbed onto the table, still wearing her London Fog, while Nurse Kane tightened the leather restraints around her wrists and ankles. As Kane turned to leave, Jennifer asked, "Who did that surgery on Ella Lu?"

Kane stopped, turned back. "It's beautiful, isn't it? And done completely without anesthesia."

Jennifer swallowed hard, couldn't answer.

"You'll meet the surgeon in the morning. But I'll give you a hint. It's somebody you know." She turned out the lights and left.

Jennifer lay awake staring up at the darkness, listening to soft moans and occasional ear-splitting shrieks from the girls nearby. Maria Ortez didn't move during the night, but slept as though she were drugged. Jennifer's mind raced, trying to think of a means of escape. And she fought with herself a thousand times to force the picture from her mind of David West carefully drilling away the bone of Ella Lu's spine and Lisa's front teeth. She thought of how his nimble fingers had opened the skull of the young boy that day in surgery. And his telling her with great excitement about applying tiny silver clips to the artery about to rupture on his patient with an aneurysm. But she refused to believe West had used his skills for such a ghoulish experimental operation, without anesthesia, on those poor frightened girls. She remembered asking him who gave him his grant for experimental surgery. West's answer hammered at her senses. "Neilson," he had said. Jennifer bit at her lower lip until she tasted blood. At length, she gave in to her overpowering suspicions and sobbed uncontrollably, unheard and unattended in the cold, dark morgue.

Early the next morning, Nurse Kane posted a sign on her reception desk saying the clinic was closed. She went straight to the lab. As she unlocked the door, Josef approached carrying a tray of food. "Set it on the counter, Josef. I'll take it in."

He did, then turned toward the back door.

"We're going to be moving," Kane said. "Take all the animals to the crematorium."

Josef said he didn't understand.

"Washington canceled all the patents on Opain. Neilson's due back tonight or tomorrow, and we'll leave. I want no trace of our work left here."

Josef frowned. "What about the patients?"

Kane picked up the tray, walked toward the rear door. "They'll be sacrificed too. For now, get rid of the animals."

Inside the morgue, Kane distributed food to each of the girls, having to shake Maria awake. Jennifer watched, unbelieving, as Kane set small portions of scrambled eggs beside each girl's head, as though feeding a tethered dog. Maria strained to suck the eggs into her mouth, swallowed noisily, and licked at the plastic plate.

"Maria," Jennifer said, almost a whisper.

Maria turned quickly to face Jennifer, her eyes wild, disoriented for an instant. "No, doctor. Not you, too."

Jennifer asked how long Maria had been here.

"Two days, I think. I very confuse."

"And Juan?" Jennifer stared directly into Maria's enormous brown eyes, level with her own from where she lay.

"Es why I came here. To help my Juan. He don' feel the pain. But they tie me. Make me hurt too."

Jennifer tried to smile. "We'll get out, Maria."

"The nurse say is only way to make Juan well. I don' wan' him feel pain like me. I hurt too much. He be okay, she say."

Jennifer took a deep breath. "He'll be fine, Maria. You too. They have to let us go."

Kane approached Jennifer, gathering up the plates. "Not hungry, Jennifer?" She took the plate of eggs away, quickly came back.

"Why?" Jennifer asked. "How can you do this?"

Kane smirked. "It's the ultimate test. We know animal tolerances for pain, Opain's effectiveness. But nobody has ever proven the absolute limit of human tolerance. We are proving Opain's ability to extend that tolerance to unheard-of levels."

"On human guinea pigs," Jennifer said, spitting out the words.

"You should be more scientific, doctor. Let me show

you what we've accomplished." Kane untied Jennifer's ankles and one wrist. She took the gun from her uniform pocket before releasing the other wrist and removing Jennifer's coat, tossing it on the table beside Maria. She led Jennifer into the main room, sat her in a large chair, and strapped her in. Jennifer watched as Lisa Waters eagerly drank something from a paper cup Kane held to her bloodstained lips. Jennifer shuddered at the sight of the wires attached to the exposed nerves of Lisa's front teeth. Kane handed Lisa a plastic control button, its cord extending to the console in front of her. Lisa immediately pressed the button, raising the numbers on the digital readout past 8, 10, 12. Lisa's body tightened and her breathing grew more rapid as the numbers passed through 16, 18, and up to 20. Jennifer heard her grunts of effort, saw the veins on her forehead bulge under her thin skin until she thought they would burst. Lisa's blue eyes seemed to grow larger, and stared unblinking at the readout straight ahead. Jennifer watched the girl's blood pressure rise to one-eighty, then one-ninety on the console's screen, her pulse rapidly escalating to one-eighty-four. "Stop," Jennifer cried. "You'll kill her."

Kane didn't move, but watched the numbers climb. "That's the point. We must know the human's viable tolerance."

Moments later, Lisa passed out, slumped down in her chair. The readout registered 28. Jennifer was drenched with perspiration, her face hot, her blood boiling.

Kane repeated a similar test with Laniet Teague. Laniet let out cries that were half-anguish, half-pleasure up to a pain level of 32, then shuddered almost orgasmically and went limp, her red hair damp and clinging to her mottled face and neck.

"You're insane," Jennifer rasped.

Kane turned back to Lisa Waters, beginning to stir. She held another cup to Lisa's lips, glanced at her watch. Moments later, she did the same for Laniet. She turned and went to the next room, then wheeled the table on which Ella Lu Mavis lay up to the pain machine.

Ella Lu rolled her large head to one side, stared at Jennifer with big accusing eyes. "They cut me," she said.

Jennifer couldn't answer. She felt the tears helplessly streaming down her face, tasted a bitter bile in her throat. Kane quickly attached pairs of wires to each of Ella Lu's exposed spinal nerves, raised the pain dial to 12, and pressed the button. Ella Lu's back arched instantly, her neck and legs raising up on the table, straining against the creaking leather restraints. Her blood pressure shot up to two-ten over one-forty, and her dark skin glistened with beads of perspiration. Kane paused for a few seconds, raised the dial to 18, and stimulated her again. At pain level 24, Ella Lu had a full-blown convulsion, a grand-mal seizure, emptying her bladder on the table as she jerked and twisted, unconscious. Jennifer screamed out as blood gushed from the girl's mouth, but Kane ignored her protests.

"That's without Opain," Kane said quietly. "With it, she went up to thirty-six."

"But she had Opain," Jennifer shrieked. "That's why her appendix ruptured. You're killing her."

Kane switched off the machine as Ella Lu twitched and jerked on the table, blood foaming from her mouth. "Her appendix is out, and her abdomen drained," Kane said. "Her infection is cured."

Jennifer shook her head. "But . . . how? Who?"

Kane walked quickly behind Jennifer, came back with a rolled-up blanket on her arm. She unrolled the blanket and laid little Juan Ortez on the counter beside the pain console, a plaster cast covering his right foot. She attached wires to needles implanted beneath his fingernails and one to his tiny penis.

Jennifer struggled against her restraints, her head pounding, her jaw clenched painfully. "No. No," was all she could force through her gritted teeth. She closed her eyes tightly, refusing to watch. Seconds later, she heard a wet, sucking sound, but no cries, no screams. When she looked, little Juan kicked his tiny brown legs and sucked at his lips almost gleefully. The digital readout registered 38. His blood pressure and pulse were normal, and he had an erection.

"That's what Opain can do," Kane said, switching off the machine.

Jennifer tried to swallow, took a deep breath. She was limp, exhausted, but her heart raced in her chest. "I don't understand," she managed.

"He feels nothing. His mother had Opain right before his birth. It crossed the placental circulation, and he got most of it."

"But it's abnormal," Jennifer protested. "He has to feel pain to survive."

Kane detached Juan from the wires. "It would wear off eventually. Or can be reversed."

"Reversed?"

Kane carried Juan off, came back. "Didn't you see the drug numbers four and five on the computer readouts you stole?"

Jennifer felt her cheeks burn again. "Yes."

"Four is oral Opain. Mixed with the hydrochloric acid in the stomach, it becomes a different compound, the chloride salt. It's a hundred times as potent as Opain by injection. That's why these patients crave severe pain. It feels good to them. We discovered that by accident, but it may be our greatest discovery. Drug number five is Antopain. Neilson wouldn't release Opain until he had a specific antagonist. Antopain totally reverses the effects of Opain."

Kane switched on the console in front of Lisa Waters. "I gave her Antopain several minutes ago. Watch." Taking the button, Lisa pressed the numbers up to 3 and screamed, throwing the control switch to the floor. Kane picked it up and pressed it again. Lisa shrieked, twisted hysterically, gave a final deep guttural gagging sound, and lost consciousness. Her blood pressure was one-ninety-four, pulse one-eighty. The digital readout showed a pain level of 10, about the same as a moderate case of shingles for the average person.

As Kane switched the machine off again, Laniet Teague began to moan. "It hurts," she said. "Bad."

"What hurts?" Kane asked.

"Everything. My arm, legs. My back. Please."

Kane ignored her, turned to Jennifer. "Well?"

Jennifer wanted to lash out at the woman, pulled at her restraints till her flesh burned. "You beast," she said. "You'll never get away with this."

Kane laughed. "You simplistic little fool. Of course we'll get away with it. By tomorrow night, most of New York City will be in the streets craving the biggest pain they can find. Crashing their cars into each other for the thrill of it. Setting themselves on fire. Breaking bones, slicing off toes, fingers, poking out their eyes. And there's only one antidote."

Jennifer couldn't follow her.

"Opain in the water supply," Kane said. "And we'll be safe and secure, well out of this country. With the only antidote to stop their suicidal madness, Antopain. It should be worth a few hundred million dollars, don't you think?"

A wave of dizziness swept over Jennifer, black spots floating before her eyes like cobwebs. She lowered her head to her chest, fighting at the edge of consciousness. Finally she looked up, spoke weakly, her voice hoarse. "Does Dr. Neilson know about this?"

Kane leaned back against the console, folded her arms. "All he needs to know," she said. "I'll tell him the rest later."

A door slammed behind Jennifer, and heavy footsteps approached her chair. She stiffened. They were the same footsteps she'd heard in the stairwell, the ones that followed her from Ella Lu's apartment, and in the tunnel before the lights went out. Kane smiled her icy smile, said, "Would you like to meet your surgeon, Jennifer? You complimented his work on Ella Lu."

Jennifer shut her eyes tightly and prayed. She couldn't bear the thought of looking up into David West's face after what she'd felt for him. She'd almost rather die than believe she could be so totally wrong.

"Open your eyes," Kane commanded. When Jennifer refused, Kane slapped her harshly across the cheek, causing her to jerk back and glare up at Kane and Josef. She quickly turned her head from side to side, looking for West, but saw nobody else. "Is this a joke?" she asked.

Josef smiled. "No joke, doctor. I'm sorry you're here." He spoke without his heavy slow drawl, and the dullness was gone from his face. His eyes were alert, intelligent. He quickly faced Nurse Kane, nodded toward Ella Lu. "What happened?"

"She convulsed again. At twenty-four."

Josef frowned, stroked his chin. "That's up from eighteen. She's developing a tolerance." He walked to Ella Lu's side, inspected his handiwork through the plastic cover, and detached the wires.

"What about the animals?" Kane asked.

"All cremated," he said, preoccupied, "except the chimps."

"Get it done, Josef. There isn't much time."

He took a paper towel from the counter, wiped the blood from Ella Lu's unconscious mouth, forced her jaw open, and looked in. "Tongue laceration," he said. "During the seizure."

"Josef!" Kane barked, her voice critical.

Without a word, he turned, glanced at Jennifer, and left the room. Jennifer stared up at Kane, unable to believe what she'd seen and heard. "Josef did that surgery?"

Kane began collecting her notebooks, pens, opened a desk drawer beneath the console. "And her appendix," Kane said. "He had his M.D. degree from UCLA, a Ph.D. from Stanford."

"Had?"

"Josef has a little problem with drugs. At one time, it was women. But he's useful."

Jennifer sat silent for a long while, watching Kane pack boxes and pile stacks of papers on the desk. Lisa and Laniet seemed to float in and out of consciousness, often groaning and sobbing in their disturbed stupor. Finally she broke her silence. "Who tried to kill me in my apartment?"

Kane didn't even look up. "Josef. But it was only to scare you off. If he'd wanted to kill you, you'd be dead."

Jennifer let her words register. "Then why the sudden change? You were almost friendly the last few days."

Kane stiffened, narrowed her eyes at Jennifer. "When you came to Frank's apartment, I knew you'd been there before. You even knew about his habit of taking the phone off the hook. I know he has a thing for younger women. But I've never known who." She paused, but her face flushed. "I wanted to keep you around. When you know your enemy, it's easier to deal with them."

Jennifer hesitated. "I wasn't after Neilson."

"Ha! You'd grab him in a minute. Especially when he's worth billions." She dropped her voice to a whisper. "You can just forget him. He's mine. Money and all." She stormed out of the room.

Minutes later, Kane returned with a hypodermic syringe in her hand. "You may as well serve some useful purpose before you die."

Jennifer tried to resist, thrusting and kicking, as Kane injected something into the vein of her right arm. Within seconds, she felt her limbs go heavy and her head begin to tilt, the room suddenly spinning before her eyes. As she fought to stay alive, she felt herself being sucked down the vortex of a whirling dark vacuum until her world went completely silent and black.

19

![decorative divider]

Jennifer awoke disoriented, uncertain of the time or where she was. She tried to move from her uncomfortable position, but nothing responded to her efforts except her head. Two gray steel bars stood upright near her face. As her mind cleared, she strained to look around her, and realized she was stripped down to panties and bra, and strapped facedown on a narrow platform inside a large animal cage like the ones she had seen for the chimpanzees. Wires extended from her fingernail beds and her nose, and when she tried to move, she felt something pull painfully deep inside her ears.

"You're finally awake," Kane said. "Drink this." She held a paper cup full of clear liquid through the bars.

Jennifer started to shake her head, felt a knifelike pain stab at her ears. "No."

Kane withdrew the cup. "Very well." She took a red rubber feeding tube from the adjacent table and stuck it into Jennifer's nose, grabbing a handful of hair with the other hand to hold her still.

Jennifer gagged when the tube touched the back of her throat, tried to spit it out with her tongue. Kane withdrew it slightly and jammed it down again, making her retch violently until bitter green slime burned her throat and dripped from her chin. Against her every

226

desire, she felt the rubber tube slide past the back of her tongue and throat, and knew it was in her esophagus.

Kane stepped back, poured the contents of the cup down the tube. "When you feel you can't live without pain, press down with your chin. The lever there will raise the pain stimulus as high as you want. Unless you die first."

Jennifer tried to squeeze the burning tears from her eyes, coughed, and tried to speak. "You bitch," she whispered. Kane wheeled around and left her view, but she could hear activity somewhere to her left. Jennifer tried her best to vomit, desperate to rid her stomach of the drug, but she couldn't make it happen. She steeled her mind to resist, not to allow her chin to press the pain lever, no matter how badly she craved the sensation. A picture of Melanie Wardner flashed before her eyes, bound and gagged in her hospital bed, thrashing against her bonds, fighting desperately for the pain she had to have. And the final picture she'd always have of Melanie, immodestly cleaved and gutted on a cold steel slab with her life's blood and juices gurgling down some impersonal drain. At least, Jennifer thought, my eyes don't sting anymore. As realization dawned, she almost drowned in a sea of panic.

"No," she screamed, struggling against her restraints. She shook her head violently, aware of only a slight tingle in her ears and the suffocating oppression of heavy straps around her back and thighs, as though the tiny cage was getting smaller, closing in around her. "No." She fought desperately for air, the stench of her own stale perspiration clogging her nostrils, her head unsteady, reeling, as an increasing vertigo spun her brain within her skull like a child's humming top. She heard a distant voice sobbing, a sad, heart-wrenching cry, and only vaguely recognized it as coming from her own throat. The next thing she knew, she felt an exciting tickle somewhere inside her ears, not unlike the numbing jolt of touching a shorted-out lamp socket, and realized her chin was pressing down hard against the lever beneath her head. The wires under her fingernails hummed like a thousand bumblebees, and tantalizing stings raced up her arms toward her brain, but not fast enough. She lunged at the lever with her chin, bringing her head down in sharp chops to make it go faster, and felt something wonderful snap and sizzle inside her nose, aware of the cauterized smell of burning flesh. Saliva drooled from her mouth as she ignored the blinking red numbers that steadily rose past 24 to 25, obsessed with her need to feel more. She bit at her tongue, tasted the metallic warmth of her own blood, but felt nothing she could enjoy. Perspiration dripped from the tip of her nose, ran down her cheeks, and angered her that it made the lever slippery, harder to get a firm grip on with her chin. She heard something pop in her neck, but strained to tighten her muscles into steel cables, to force the high keening noise in her ears to penetrate her brain, or shatter her skull like a crystal goblet. Yes, she thought. Shatter and explode, with a mushroom cloud of vaporized brain to drink in the white-hot heat and savor the deep thunder of the blast. Blood trickled from one side of her nose, felt sticky on the lever under her chin. A series of thrills undulated up her spine in onrushing waves, as when somebody walks over your grave, and she felt her back muscles spasm into a thousand knotted snakes while something creaked and popped in her spine. A kaleidoscope of brilliant colors suddenly burst before her eyes, flashing, blinding, sputtering at the edges like night fireworks on the fourth of July. Something red burned the number 31 through the glare just as a series of a hundred successive orgasms racked her body and paralyzed her mind. "David," she cried. "Oh, yes, David. More." The brightest white light she had ever seen flared in her eyes, silent, and she fell limp, unconscious—a rag doll tied and tortured by a twisted child, its button eyes plucked out, abandoned in a monkey's cage.

Jennifer awoke late that afternoon, her body aching as though she had been autopsied and put back together. The nerves and muscles in her neck screamed at her as she tried to raise her head. She felt the rubber tube slide up and out her nose.

"Are you all right?" Dr. Neilson asked.

Jennifer strained to focus her eyes on his blurred figure, couldn't respond.

"I've given you Antopain," he said. "When you're able, I'll help you out of the cage."

Jennifer painfully turned her head to watch Neilson force Lisa and Laniet to drink something he offered, his voice calm and reassuring as he spoke to each of them. He poured a small quantity of the clear liquid into a baby bottle and put the nipple in Juan Ortez's mouth, propping the bottle on a pillow. Jennifer slowly moved one hand up to her face, felt for the wires at her nose and ears. They were gone, as were her restraints.

"Es to be okay, doctor. He a good man."

Jennifer turned to Maria, sitting up on the table beside the cage, smiling, but rubbing her wrists. "He help my Juan. You see."

Neilson quickly approached Jennifer again, virtually lifted her from the animal cage, and helped her to a chair. His face was flushed, his brow soaked, and his eyes distant and cold. Nurse Kane was nowhere in sight. Without a word, Neilson rummaged through a desk drawer, withdrew a hammer, and began beating first one, then another pain-machine console to smithereens. He smashed two glass bottles resting on a counter, spilling their clear liquid contents onto the linoleum floor. Jennifer stared, wide-eyed, as he opened a metal cabinet and dumped box after box of glass vials on the floor, stomping them with his feet in his rage until no single vial remained intact. He bolted through the open door, hammer in hand, like a madman, the sound of smashing glass, splintering wood, and ripping metal marking his destructive path. Jennifer tried to rise from her chair, but began to black out again, and fell back, lowering her head to her shaking knees. Maria used the opportunity to run to her baby and gather him up, quickly bringing him back to the table beside Jennifer. Lisa Waters and Laniet Teague began to move around where they sat in their torture chairs, their eyes open and wide, frightened and questioning. Elle Lu Mavis lay perfectly still, facing the floor, apparently unconscious. The wires had been removed from her exposed spine.

Jennifer finally managed to speak, her voice thick and raspy, foreign to her own ears. "Got to get out," she said.

Maria huddled Juan closer to her body, her brown eyes darting around the room, uncertain where to hide. She didn't move.

Minutes later, Neilson reappeared, his white dress shirt soaked under his arms and clinging to his back. His face was tense, his jaw firmly set, and his eyes reddened, enraged. "Where is Kane?" he demanded.

Jennifer shook her head. Maria stared silently down at her baby, rocked him back and forth in her arms.

Jennifer tried to clear her throat. "You didn't know?"

He raised the hammer as though it had grown to his clenched fist. "This . . . this inhumanity?" He growled with contempt, disgust. "Never," he said, a muscle at the corner of his mouth twitching as he glared at Jennifer. "Human experiments, yes. But not this savagery."

Jennifer tried to rise again, made it only by holding to the chair for support. "Then I'm leaving."

Neilson reached to take her arm.

"Stop right there," Nurse Kane shouted. "What in hell are you doing?"

Jennifer quickly looked behind Neilson as he turned. Kane stood beside Josef with gun in hand, her eyes wild and frenzied. Neilson raised the hammer and pointed it at her. "How could you?" he demanded.

"Put the hammer down, Franklyn. You'll thank me when you see the results. Opain is perfect. And Antopain."

He paled, his voice shook when he answered. "Opain is to stop suffering, not create it. What you've done is a sacrilege."

"What we've done is prove beyond any doubt that it works in humans, virtually abolishes the viable tolerance level. With Opain, humans can withstand unheard-of amounts of pain and survive."

"What about her?" Neilson shouted, nodding toward Ella Lu.

Kane glared coldly back at Neilson. "She withstood pain more severe than ever recorded, on every single sensory nerve in her body. A thousand times worse than any pain known to man."

Neilson took a step toward Ella Lu. "And she's dead."

Kane's eyes flickered briefly. "Because I reversed the Opain. Without it, she couldn't bear the smallest stimulus."

Josef quickly walked to Ella Lu's lifeless body, felt her neck and wrist, scanned her open spinal cord. He brushed a greenish-black fly off her head and turned to Kane. "You didn't tell me."

She ignored him, spoke to Neilson. "There's still time, Frank. We can go to Brazil, Europe. Anywhere. It's worth hundreds of millions."

Neilson's shoulders slumped. "After this? Murder?"

"Nobody will know. We'll cremate them. There'll be no trace."

Neilson's voice dropped to a husky whisper, a tremor audible when he spoke. "We'll go nowhere, Rachael. I will start over. But not with you." He turned, took Jennifer's arm. "Come on," he said.

Kane flipped the safety off the automatic pistol. "After what I've done for you? I sacrificed the last ten years waiting for you. I ignored your little flings. The young sweet things you couldn't keep your hands off. But no more. We're in this together, and I'll swear to it. We'll take our Opain and get out. Nobody has it but us."

"The Chinese have it."

Kane smirked. "Don't be such a fool. I filled some vials with morphine sulfate, labeled them 'Opain.' That's what you gave the Chinese. You can't trust them. We have the Opain, Frank. You and me."

Neilson almost laughed, an ironic sound. "There is no Opain, Rachael. I destroyed it. All of it. And Antopain." He stopped for an instant, lowered his voice. "Do you know why I needed those young girls? Because you turned into an old hag. A nagging, demanding, domineering old hag. I let you convince me we deserved to be rich. To live like billionaires. Now I see that's all you ever wanted. You didn't give a damn about people. Their suffering." He tugged at Jennifer's arm, nodded toward Maria. "Let's get out of here."

"Not with her," Kane said in a voice as dead and cold as dry ice. She raised the gun toward Jennifer and fired just as Neilson lunged forward. Jennifer recoiled, fell back in her chair holding her ears, the sudden smell of gunpowder in the air. Neilson took three lurching steps toward Kane and fell, clutching his throat as his hammer clattered to the floor beside him. His legs jerked convulsively for an instant, and then he was still. Jennifer screamed, leaped from her chair toward where Neilson lay. Josef jumped toward her, grabbed her arms. "Don't," he said quietly, turning her around and forcing her back to her seat.

Josef immediately went to Neilson's side, turned him over, and felt for his carotid pulse. He looked up, first at Jennifer, then at Nurse Kane, her gun lowered to her side. "He's dead." Josef stood, walked slowly toward Kane. Maria sobbed beside Jennifer. Lisa and Laniet stared from their chairs with anxious eyes, strapped in place, their faces unbelieving, their lips so tightly pressed together they blanched.

Kane immediately raised her gun, aimed it at Josef, a look of desperation on her face. "There's still all that money, Josef. I have the formula."

He took another step. "And you'd take me?"

"Of course. You can still do your surgery. The experiments. We'll buy you a license in another country."

He stopped, dropped his hands to his sides, working the muscles in his jaw.

"And the heroin, Josef. I still have plenty of heroin."

Josef shook his head, clenched and unclenched his fists repeatedly. "I've got to get cured," he whispered. "Somehow."

"I'll help you," Kane said. "I promise."

Josef straightened, took a deep breath. Finally he made his decision. He nodded.

Kane visibly relaxed. "Carry him to the crematorium, Josef. I'll take care of things here."

Josef lifted Neilson's body from the floor. Jennifer saw a tiny puncture wound in the midline of Neilson's throat, with virtually no blood around it. The bullet must have gone straight through his trachea into his cervical spine, she thought. A painless, instant death. As Josef carried the body from the room, Kane turned to Jennifer, gun in hand. "You caused him to turn against me," Kane said. The gun trembled in her hand as badly as her voice, and her eyes filled with tears.

Jennifer gripped the arms of her chair. She didn't speak.

Kane grabbed two of the restraints from the cage and fastened them around Jennifer's wrists, securing them to the arms of the wooden chair. She ordered Maria to lie down and tied her wrists as well, Maria screaming and kicking when she pulled Juan away and put him on the floor. Kane quickly checked Lisa and Laniet's restraints and left the room. Moments later, she returned with three metal cans, opened them, and sloshed their smelly contents throughout the room. Jennifer recognized the strong aroma of ether immediately, the most flammable of all anesthetic agents, worse than gasoline.

"You can't do this," Jennifer said.

Kane stopped for an instant, glared at her. "Your death won't be painless, you little whore. I want you to feel every flame that licks at your shapely legs, burns away your pretty young face a piece at a time. Maybe *he* didn't want me, but others will." Kane worked frantically, desperate, as she spoke. "Money is what buys love, you fool. Not youth. I've waited ten years for this. And I won't be cheated now." She hurried out the door, pulled it almost shut, and threw in a lighted match, slamming the door as the room burst into flames.

Jennifer strained at her bonds until they cut into her raw flesh, unable to hear her own desperate grunts of effort for the shrieks and wails of Maria and the other two girls. The stench of ether was quickly replaced by an overwhelming heat from the leaping flames filling the room. Black smoke rose in the air as the wooden counter and a table ignited, and something sputtered near the pain machine, like a fallen power line in a storm, adding the smell of burned electrical wiring. Maria screamed in Spanish, Jennifer able to understand only the name Juan among her hysterical shouts. The sound of voices shouting beyond the door penetrated an instant of desperate silence, and two shots followed in rapid succession. A great tongue of bluish-yellow flame leaped up on Jennifer's right, singeing her hair and stinging her cheek, causing her to kick violently with her unbound feet. Her chair balanced precariously for a second, then toppled to her left, crashing her to the floor, striking her arm painfully as she heard a sickening snap, certain her arm had fractured. She fought to recover her senses, and twisted and pulled with all her might against the restraints, her mind racing, her desperate eyes fixed on the hungry flames advancing steadily, unrelenting, across the floor toward where she lay. Suddenly her left wrist broke free, a splintered piece of the chair's arm dangling in the leather strap. Fighting furiously against time and heat she clawed at the strap on her right wrist as a towering wall of flames ignited the ceiling, rapidly engulfing the room, consuming everything in its path. The instant her wrist broke free, she grabbed little Juan from the floor and struggled to her feet, her limbs stiff and painful, but somehow strengthened by the adrenaline surging through her body.

"Maria," she screamed, untying the hysterical woman's arms as she lay shrieking in Spanish, her head violently shaking from side to side, eyes squeezed tightly shut. Jennifer slapped her face sharply, pulled her upright, and shoved her baby into her arms. As Maria clutched her child to her breast and moaned, rocking him back and forth, Jennifer grabbed up her raincoat and used it as a shield to dash through a fleeting gap in the advancing wall of flames. She stumbled over something and lurched toward where Lisa screamed, almost crashing headlong into her chair. She untied Lisa with reckless abandon, hardly aware of the searing heat of the metal buckles on her fingers. A great yellow ball of flames whooshed and billowed toward her face for an instant, its explosive intensity knocking her back, almost to the floor. Lisa grabbed at her arm as she struggled to get to Laniet, her eyes stinging, trying to force themselves shut against the dense smoke. She fought to stop a spasm of rib-twisting coughs as she saw Laniet Teague's red hair burst into flames and her skin char and melt before her blurring eyes. The girl's body was half-consumed, engulfed in flames and greasy smoke, and what was left of her head hung limply on her chest. Jennifer forced Lisa to the floor, her coat over their heads, and raced on hands and bloody knees back toward Maria's wailing prayers. She finally saw Maria, huddled on the floor in the back corner, her eyes wide and frenzied, her face that of a fox trapped in a forest fire, her pup to her breast.

Jennifer grabbed at a hot handle on the bank of small square doors, the old storage racks for corpses, and shoved Lisa toward the dark interior. "Get in," she yelled, and grabbed Maria's arm, dragging her toward the door. Maria resisted blindly, but finally scampered inside. Jennifer lunged through the opening and slammed the door behind just as a ceiling lamp exploded and showered the door with white sparks and fragments of flying glass.

Breathless, Jennifer sat back against the door and coughed till she almost threw up. Water streamed from her burning eyes, and the smell of singed human hair and flesh clung to her nostrils. Maria wept somewhere in the dark and dank cave, the only sound audible above her own gasping breaths. Jennifer leaned her head against the door, limp with exhaustion, and took a long breath of the welcome musty but cool air.

"Oh, God," Lisa whined. "We're trapped."

Jennifer tried to force her eyes to adjust to the darkness, but it was no use. The black surrounding them was the black of an ancient grave, untouched for years by the faintest light. "Somebody will find us," she said. "And we're insulated against the fire."

"But we'll suffocate," Lisa said in her small voice.

Jennifer tried to remember how many doors she had seen stacked into the wall. Eight? Twelve? She knew the interior of the storage compartment should be one large chamber, designed to refrigerate all the bodies with one cooling unit. "There's plenty of air, Lisa." Mildewy and stale, she thought, but better than the conflagration outside.

After a long silence, broken only by Maria's wet sniffs, Lisa asked, "Is this where they keep dead people?"

Jennifer hesitated. "It's where *we* stay alive."

They sat silently for an indeterminable time, frightened, waiting, listening. Maria finally got control of herself, said she was okay. The insulated door that kept out the fire also kept out all sound, so they had no way of knowing what was happening outside. Jennifer didn't dare open the door from the storage rack to find out. It would take several hours for the fire to die down unless somebody spotted it and put it out. Surely they'll see the smoke, she thought. Please let somebody see the smoke. Jennifer began to feel hot and stuffy, felt perspiration trickle down the sides of her chest and forehead. She groped blindly to her side, identified the sliding steel rack above and below that had cooled and preserved countless corpses before the new morgue was built. She debated crawling over the racks to see what had happened outside. She unbuttoned the top of her blouse, felt something tickle as it ran down her chest.

"It's like an oven in here," Lisa said. "I can't breathe."

"Stay calm," Jennifer said quietly. "You'll use up less oxygen."

Another long silence followed. After about an hour of the increasing heat and oppressive quarters, Jennifer heard an unmistakable wet sucking sound. "Maria?" she asked. "Is that Juan?"

"I feedin' my son," Maria replied. "He get hungry."

Jennifer felt the tension lessen immediately, made her decision. She told the others to stay where they were while she checked. It was slow going, crawling to the far end of the cooler, and she scraped her shins and bumped her head on the metal racks. At last she felt a solid wall ahead of her, knew she was near the front of the room. She fumbled in the dark for the door latch. The inside of the heavy door was not too hot to touch, but had heated up considerably. She felt where she knew a latch should be, felt again. She checked the opposite side of the door's interior. It was perfectly smooth. Panic welled up inside her as she ran her hands over the door's surface from top to bottom and back again. Her pulse hammered in her ears. There has to be an inside latch, she told herself, searching again. But it wasn't there. She quickly felt her way back to the adjacent rack, running her hands across that door. Nothing. She pushed against the door with both hands, straining. It wouldn't budge. My God, she thought. We're trapped. And nobody will ever know we were here. It could be years before anybody opens one of these doors. She crouched on her knees and blindly searched the doors above. The same. Overwhelmed by a sense of futility, she sat back on her feet and dropped her head to her hands, tears silently streaming down her hot face.

"What's wrong?" Lisa asked, her voice hollow, echoing through the metal chamber. "Won't it open?"

Jennifer forced herself to straighten, swallowed hard. "The door's still warm," she said. "I'm going to wait." She searched her mind frantically. There had to be a way out. Stupid, stupid, she thought. Of course they wouldn't put handles on the inside of body-storage doors. Who would ever need to get out? She imagined some innocent janitor opening the chamber someday and finding the semiclothed skeletons of three women and a baby. She wondered if they'd bother to try to identify them. She wondered if David would ever know how she died. If he would care, or even remember. She felt she had to tell Lisa and Maria, but knew she wouldn't. They'd only panic, become hysterical, and hasten their deaths. If she could keep them calm, they'd simply lapse into a coma from oxygen starvation and go to sleep.

Juan first, because of his higher metabolism, full stomach and all. Jennifer prayed Maria would be unconscious before he died. As that picture settled on her mind, Jennifer snapped her head up, forced her eyes open wide in the dark, and took several giant breaths to force the dizziness and impending lassitude from her brain. She shifted her body until she sat facing the blank door and braced her arms behind her. Coiling her knees under her chin, she heaved both feet at the heavy door, jarring her brain more awake from the impact. She vaguely heard Lisa's voice ask something in the hollow distance as she pulled her legs back and struck out again. She reached above her head for better support, grasped the sides of the upper body rack, causing it to roll slightly forward on its wheeled track, clanging noisily against the upper door. With the combination of arm and leg thrusts, she battered both doors with a savage fury, trying to ignore the webs of unconsciousness settling on the edges of her mind. She would have screamed when something touched her shoulder, like a finger bone rotted of its flesh, but her protective reflexes had dipped deeper into that atavistic well and drove her on with the most basic of all urges, the blind determination to survive.

"I help," Maria said, settling herself into position beside Jennifer and picking up the rhythm of her thrusts.

The heavy door rattled and thumped, promised to give way at first, but seemed to grow stronger as they tired, denying its promise, as though personally antagonistic, refusing them freedom from their entombment as it had to others so many times before.

"But we're not dead," Jennifer yelled at the door, and kicked again.

She stopped for a moment to catch her faltering breath, heard Maria gasping beside her. She was drenched through and through, limp, her heart racing to pump dark blood to her fading brain. Her lungs screamed out for air. Suddenly a wail of protest assaulted her ears, an infant's cry echoing through the black tomb.

"My baby," Maria rasped, stiffening beside Jennifer.

Lisa's tiny voice answered as he interrupted his cry for breath. "It's okay. He's only wet."

Maria clutched Jennifer's arm, her nails digging into her flesh. "He feel, doctor. My baby cried. He gonna be okay."

Jennifer immediately grasped the metal rack above her and thrust her feet against the door again, mustering a final ounce of strength from some unknown reservoir. The room beyond the door might be a blazing inferno, certain to cremate them immediately or bake them well done in death's oven in which they lay. But she had to try. She couldn't give up. Her joints creaked and ached, and her muscles screamed for relief as the door suddenly burst open.

20

———◆◆◆———

"What the hell?" a man shouted. "Get some oxygen over here."

Jennifer felt somebody pull at her feet, sliding the body rack into the beam of a flashlight. A hand took her arm and sat her up. Seconds later, a rubber mask covered her nose and mouth, and she sucked in great hungry breaths of clean air. She pulled the mask down against rough hands and tried to shout, but heard herself barely whisper, "Up there. A woman and a baby." Somebody stood her up and supported her on a strong arm as she stumbled toward the door.

"I told you before, doc, get back," a harsh voice shouted.

"Fuck off," David West bellowed, pushing past the burly fireman. "Jennie. Sweetheart. You all right?" He grabbed Jennifer around the waist, walked her to the outside corridor, and sat her against the wall. Silent tears streamed down his cheeks as he knelt beside her, brushing her singed hair off her face. She saw the others being helped out the door, pulled David close against her, and cried.

When she awoke that evening, alone in David's bed, Jennifer got up and slowly walked to the bathroom. She turned on the light, supporting herself on the sink while she studied her smudged face and singed hair and eyebrows. West's face appeared behind her in the mirror, and he silently slipped his arms around her waist.

"I never knew it was possible to be so sore," she said.

He grinned his flashing grin. "I'll massage you." He took her hand and directed her into the bedroom. "I've got something for you," he said, turning on the bedroom light.

"Goldfish," she said, stooping to look straight into the side of the bowl on his dresser. One large and one small fringetail goldfish stared silently back at her, mouths working. "Oh, David, they're beautiful."

"The big one gets all the food," he said. "You have to put them in separate bowls to feed them."

She jumped up and hugged him. "Thank you, David." As she turned to walk beside him, she asked, "Who's the little boy in those pictures?" She nodded toward the framed photographs resting on the bedside table.

"My little brother," he said.

She didn't understand. "But you said you were an orphan."

"I am," he said. "I help out with an organization called Big Brothers. It's for kids without fathers."

Jennifer walked over and picked up one photo. A blond youth of about ten with wary blue eyes stared out at her. "That's where you were all those nights you were busy?"

He nodded. "And on weekends."

She threw her arms around him and pulled him tight against her, unable to believe that she had even fleetingly considered him capable of anything sinister. "There's so much about you I don't know," she said. "Why didn't you tell me?"

West took the photo from her. "Orphans get in the habit of not opening up to people. Like him." He set the photograph back on the table, smiled. "I'm trying to teach him something I'm still learning myself."

"And I want to know everything about you, David West."

West kissed the top of her head. "Chinese or pizza?" he asked.

She wiped a tear from her cheek and turned her face up to his. "Something cold."

Over a cold antipasto and bottle of chilled Soave that evening, Jennifer and David discussed the details of her experience.

"I came looking for you," he said. "When you didn't answer your phone or your page, I remembered what you'd said about having a key to the back rooms. I couldn't find Nurse Kane or Neilson, so I tried to get in the rear of the lab. That's when I smelled the smoke. I called the fire department, and they cut through the doors with axes. God, Jennie, I died every time they brought out another body. I couldn't be sure."

"Did they find Kane? Neilson?"

West shook his head. "Who knows? They were all beyond recognition. Mostly charred bones. There were four human bodies altogether. And one chimp."

Jennifer counted in her head, stiffened. "David, there should have been five. Neilson, Ella Lu, Laniet Teague, Josef, and Kane."

West frowned. "The firemen said four. And a chimp. They were certain."

Jennifer stood, walked to the window, stared out at a sleeting rain and glistening cars below. She pulled her robe tighter around her, hugged her arms to her chest. "Then somebody got away." She turned to see West's questioning face staring back at her, his wineglass halted in midair.

"Kane?" he said.

"Or Josef. I heard shots from the other room after Kane started the fire."

"You said Kane had the gun. She must have shot Josef and put him in the crematorium."

Jennifer shuddered. "Or they struggled, and he shot her. Oh, God, David. Pray Kane didn't get away. She knows the Opain formula. And there's no Antopain to reverse it."

Without another word, West picked up the phone and called the police. When they came, Jennifer told them everything she knew. Two detectives from Homicide joined the officers, agreed to put out an APB on Nurse Kane and Josef, and asked Jennifer to come by the station the next day.

When the policemen left, she curled up on the sofa against West. "Can you imagine what could happen if Kane sold the formula to another country? They'd have the power to drive entire cities mad. A few gallons in the water supply of any city in the world, and the people would literally self-destruct, searching for ways to feel pain."

"Worse yet, what if Neilson had sold Opain to the Chinese?"

Jennifer raised her head from his shoulder. "Why are they any worse than anybody else? What about Russia? Iran?"

"Which country would benefit most from an all-out thermonuclear war, Jennie? If Russia and the U.S. were both suddenly drugged with Opain, not only the citizens but also the men who have the authority to push the big button would be crazy to feel more pain. Somebody would push that button. And China is the only country with a population big enough to survive the holocaust. We'd be wiped out. China would still have a few million people left. They'd take over the world."

Jennifer sipped her wine, set it down. "That's a bit farfetched, David. Even if it is true. I think Kane would be more likely to sell it to the Arabs. She'd go where the biggest money is. Then they'd have all the oil and all the Opain. People would pay more any day to keep from hurting than they would for gasoline. They'd *own* the world. It's better than taking it over."

West pulled her closer. "It was probably Josef who got away. All he'd want is his next fix, from what you say."

Jennifer thought for a moment. "No, I think he'd go in for a cure after what happened. Kane kept him hooked. I could hear it in his voice. He knew she had used him. Just as she used Neilson and everybody else. I feel sorry for Josef, in spite of what he did to Ella Lu. A brilliant man hiding behind the cloak of a dumb lab janitor for years. Cleaning out cages, sweeping the floors, whatever Kane ordered. All for a chance to do his experiments. His surgery." She shook her head. "And he was good. Perverted, but good. What a waste." She paused. "You know what was wrong with Opain? It was too damned good. Somebody would always find a way to abuse it."

In the morning, Jennifer scrambled eggs and made toast while West called to get another resident to cover for him for the day. After breakfast, she insisted on a walk before they went to the police station. She brushed the soot off her London Fog as best she could and walked out into a bright, crisp morning arm-in-arm with David. They talked and walked leisurely down to the East River, stopping frequently to kiss and to enjoy the glorious day.

"It's good to be alive," Jennifer said. "To breathe fresh air."

"What will you do now?" West asked. "The pain clinic's closed."

She paused to lean on the railing, stared into the river, watched a tug go by. "I have a job waiting in Atlanta. If I ever get my fellowship."

West picked up a stone and threw it into the river. "Still afraid of going into practice?"

She thought for a moment before answering. "No. I'm ready."

"What changed it for you?"

Jennifer watched a fish rise quickly to the top of the water and suck in a piece of flotsam. "I'm not sure exactly when I knew. So much has happened." A thousand scenes flashed before her eyes. "Maybe it was when little Juan Ortez cried out in the morgue. Or seeing Lisa Waters' eyes pleading for help." She took a deep breath.

"I knew I didn't have all the answers, but I knew more about where we were than they did."

West tossed another stone and waited.

"I know I'll never be perfect, David. I can accept that now. But if I know a little bit more about people's bodies than they do—about disease, medicines, even pain—then I have to help them the best I can. Even if I fail, I have to try."

After a long silence, West spoke. "Patients in New York need good reconstructive surgeons too."

She watched a sea gull dive to snatch something from the water and fly off, swerving and veering to stay just out of reach of three sea gulls behind him, trying to steal his catch. She silently cheered for the one who escaped and flew away, his meal intact.

West persisted. "I hear there's an opening at NYU."

Jennifer took a great lungful of the sea air, wondered if he meant what she hoped he did. "I like New York," she said.

West took her shoulders gently, turned her to face him. "Jennie, we've only known each other a short time. But I've known since our first night together. And when I thought you were dead, I couldn't live with myself. I love you, Jennie. I don't want to lose you."

She flew into his arms, happier than she could remember being in her entire life, and found his hungry, searching lips. She buried her head against his chest, squeezed him to her. "I love you, David. I think I always have."

He kissed her nose, her eyelids, her cheeks. "We'll move your things over today." He paused for an instant, tilted her face up to his. "If you're not comfortable that way, we'll get married first. Whatever you say."

She snuffled, brushed a tear from the corner of one eye. "Doesn't matter," she said, laughing. "Just so we're together." She turned to look at the water flowing by, West's arm tightly around her waist. After a moment she asked, "Who's the pretty brunette nurse you have lunch with?"

"Sarah?"

Jennifer didn't answer. She stared straight ahead.

West laughed, turned her to face him. "Sarah coordinates the Big Brother program at the hospital. She gets doctors to spend time with the kids."

"Then there's nothing between you?"

"No." He laughed again. "Hey. I think you were jealous." When Jennifer didn't answer, he continued. "She's engaged to one of my best friends." He kissed the tip of her nose, still grinning.

A freshening breeze swept off the river, biting at Jennifer's cheeks and ears. David raised the collar of his sheepskin coat.

"Cold?" he asked.

She shook her head. "I need my scarf, that's all." She reached into her coat pocket, pulled out her brown scarf, and stopped, frozen in place. "Oh, no," she groaned. Wrapped in a fold of the scarf was a glass vial. She pulled it free, held it up for David to see. Printed in bright blue letters on the glass was one word: "OPAIN." Her eyes darted from the vial to West's astonished face and back again. Her voice came out in a whisper. "My God, David. It isn't over." She suddenly remembered jamming the vial into her pocket when Kane caught her in the lab, held the gun on her.

Two vertical furrows deepened in West's brow. "That's about a billion dollars you're holding."

Jennifer swallowed hard. "The end of suffering? Or the beginning?"

West stared silently back at her, his dark eyes flashing, his face intense. The hum of morning traffic droned somewhere in the distance. A car's horn sounded, muted, far away. Water sloshed against the sea wall below the walk.

Without a word, Jennifer spun around and hurled the glass vial as far as she could throw it, into the middle of the East River. She watched the tiny splash it made, saw it sink out of sight. She put her scarf around her head, tied it tightly.

West let out a long breath, grinned his lazy grin. "How's it feel to throw away a billion dollars?"

Jennifer put her arm through his, turned to walk home. "I didn't feel a thing."

21

Jennifer raced across First Avenue in the muggy August heat of late afternoon, took the elevator up to their new apartment. Inside, she threw her arms around her husband's neck and told him the good news. "I got the job, David. At NYU. With my very own office. I'm a real reconstructive surgeon."

West hugged her close, kissed her, and backed away just enough to read the letter she waved in her hand. "Fantastic, sweetheart. Let's celebrate. I'll order in Chinese and a bottle of champagne."

"Pizza," she said, grinning. "And Valpolicella." She danced to the antique English sofa and plopped on the cushions, hugging the precious letter to her chest. "Pizza *and* Chinese," she said. She looked up at West, her face beaming. "Dreams do come true, David. I've never been happier in my life."

West poured two glasses of Chablis, toasted her good news, and picked up the phone. Jennifer flipped on the TV set while he placed their order, half-listened to the six-o'clock news.

Seconds later, she grasped David's arm hard, jumped up, and raised the TV's volume, her face rapidly draining of color.

West frowned quizzically, hung up the phone. "Jennie, what's wrong?"

"Shh," she said. "Listen."

The newscaster's voice filled the suddenly tense room. ". . . and sales of over-the-counter pain medications have mysteriously dropped in that tiny country despite an incredible rise of serious accidents and injuries. Government hospitals are so overburdened with an epidemic of burns, fractures, and knife wounds that patients will have to be evacuated to hospitals on adjacent islands or to the mainland. Prince Faoul Rashouk, of Saudi Arabia, who has a palatial retreat on the idyllic island, has volunteered to provide emergency air transport for the afflicted natives, to hospitals in his country. According to experts brought in by Prince Rashouk, a rancid form of betel nut commonly chewed on the island is responsible for the outbreak. Now, turning to the local news and weather . . ."

Jennifer turned the set off, stood staring at David, her face blank, unmoving, as if in shock. Water dripped steadily from the kitchen faucet into the sink's drain. A New York City bus sounded its horn somewhere below. Its air brakes hissed, and it roared away. She saw David's Adam's apple move when he swallowed, silent, his gaze locked on hers. Jennifer drew a deep breath, a half-sigh, felt her nails dig painfully into her palms. "Kane," she whispered, starting for the phone. "She got away."

That same afternoon, a white Lear jet roared down a shimmering hot runway on a tiny island in the Caribbean and took off. Inside, a uniformed steward entered the main cabin, bowed to the two passengers, and said, "Your drinks, sir."

Prince Faoul Rashouk nodded, his face dark beneath his white robe. He extended a bejeweled hand and passed a silver goblet of wine to his guest. As the steward bowed again and walked away, Prince Rashouk raised his glass in a toast. "You have turned the island into a most convincing laboratory, doctor. You were absolutely right about Opain. It works."

Josef smiled a perfect white smile, loosened his tie. He nodded confidently, raised his own goblet. "To pain," he said.

Prince Rashouk grinned. "Yes, doctor," he said. "To pain."